T0226926

INTERVENTIONAL CARDIOLOGY CLINICS

www.interventional.theclinics.com

Editor-in-Chief

MATTHEW J. PRICE

Intravascular Physiology

October 2015 • Volume 4 • Number 4

Editor

ALLEN JEREMIAS

ELSEVIER

1600 John F. Kennedy Boulevard • Suite 1800 • Philadelphia, Pennsylvania, 19103-2899

http://www.theclinics.com

INTERVENTIONAL CARDIOLOGY CLINICS Volume 4, Number 4
October 2015 ISSN 2211-7458, ISBN-13: 978-0-323-40090-9

Editor: Adrianne Brigido
Developmental Editor: Barbara Cohen-Kligerman

Interventional Cardiology Clinics (ISSN 2211-7458) is published quarterly by Elsevier Inc., 360 Park Avenue South, New York, NY 10010-1710. Months of issue are January, April, July, and October. Subscription prices are USD 195 per year for US individuals, USD 305 for US institutions, USD 130 per year for US students, USD 230 per year for Canadian individuals, USD 375 for Canadian institutions, USD 150 per year for Canadian students, USD 295 per year for international individuals, USD 375 for international institutions, and USD 150 per year for international students. To receive student/resident rate, orders must be accompanied by name of affiliated institution, date of term, and the *signature* of program/residency coordinator on institution letterhead. Orders will be billed at individual rate until proof of status is received. Foreign air speed delivery is included in all *Clinics* subscription prices. All prices are subject to change without notice. **POSTMASTER:** Send address changes to *Interventional Cardiology Clinics*, Elsevier Health Sciences Division, Subscription Customer Service, 3251 Riverport Lane, Maryland Heights, MO 63043. **Customer Service: Telephone: 1-800-654-2452** (U.S. and Canada); **1-314-447-8871** (outside U.S. and Canada). **Fax: 1-314-447-8029. E-mail: journalscustomerservice-usa@elsevier.com (for print support); journalsonlinesupport-usa@elsevier.com (for online support).**

Reprints. For copies of 100 or more of articles in this publication, please contact the Commercial Reprints Department, Elsevier Inc., 360 Park Avenue South, New York, NY 10010-1710. Tel.: 212-633-3874; Fax: 212-633-3820; E-mail: reprints@elsevier.com.

CONTRIBUTORS

EDITOR-IN-CHIEF

MATTHEW J. PRICE, MD
Assistant Professor, Scripps Translational
Science Institute; Director of the Cardiac
Catheterization Laboratory, Scripps Green
Hospital, La Jolla, California

EDITOR

ALLEN JEREMIAS, MD, MSc, FACC
Division of Cardiovascular Medicine,
Department of Medicine, Stony Brook
University Medical Center, Stony Brook,
New York

AUTHORS

SUNG GYUN AHN, MD, PhD
Division of Cardiology, Department of
Medicine, Emory University School of
Medicine, Atlanta, Georgia; Division of
Cardiology, Yonsei University, Wonju
College of Medicine, Yonsei University,
Seoul, Korea

LOHENDRAN BASKARAN, MD
Department of Radiology, Dalio Institute of
Cardiovascular Imaging, New York-
Presbyterian Hospital, Weill Cornell Medical
College, New York, New York

ADAM J. BROWN, MD
Department of Cardiovascular Medicine,
University of Cambridge, Cambridge,
United Kingdom

CHRISTOPHER J. BROYD, PhD, MBBS
Cardiovascular Institute, Hospital Clínico San
Carlos, Madrid, Spain

ENRICO CERRATO, MD
Cardiovascular Institute, Hospital Clínico San
Carlos, Madrid, Spain

IBRAHIM DANAD, MD
Department of Radiology, Dalio Institute of
Cardiovascular Imaging, New York-
Presbyterian Hospital, Weill Cornell Medical
College, New York, New York

JUSTIN DAVIES, BSc, MBBS, MRCP, PhD
Consultant Cardiologist and Senior Lecturer,
International Centre for Circulatory Health,
National Heart and Lung Institute, Imperial
College London, London, United Kingdom

MAURO ECHAVARRIA-PINTO, MD
Cardiovascular Institute, Hospital Clínico San
Carlos, Madrid, Spain

JAVIER ESCANED, MD, PhD
Cardiovascular Institute, Hospital Clínico San
Carlos and Universidad Complutense of
Madrid, Madrid, Spain

WILLIAM F. FEARON, MD
Professor of Medicine; Director of
Interventional Cardiology, Division of
Cardiovascular Medicine, Stanford University
Medical Center, Stanford University School of
Medicine, Stanford, California

DON P. GIDDENS, PhD
Professor of Biomedical Engineering and Dean
Emeritus, Wallace H. Coulter Department of
Biomedical Engineering, Georgia Institute of
Technology, Atlanta, Georgia

K. LANCE GOULD, MD
Martin Bucksbaum Distinguished Professor of
Medicine, Division of Cardiology,
Weatherhead PET Center for Preventing and
Reversing Atherosclerosis, Memorial Hermann
Hospital, University of Texas Medical School
at Houston, Houston, Texas

OLIVIA Y. HUNG, MD, PhD
Division of Cardiology, Department of
Medicine, Emory University School of
Medicine, Atlanta, Georgia

ALLEN JEREMIAS, MD, MSc, FACC
Division of Cardiovascular Medicine,
Department of Medicine, Stony Brook
University Medical Center, Stony Brook,
New York

NILS P. JOHNSON, MD, MS, FACC
Associate Professor of Medicine, Division of
Cardiology, Weatherhead PET Center for
Preventing and Reversing Atherosclerosis,
Memorial Hermann Hospital, University of
Texas Medical School at Houston, Houston,
Texas

MORTON J. KERN, MD
Associate Chief of Cardiology, University of
California, Irvine Medical Center, Orange,
California; Chief of Medicine, Long Beach
Veterans Affairs Medical Center, Long Beach,
California

RICHARD L. KIRKEEIDE, PhD
Associate Professor of Medicine, Division of
Cardiology, Weatherhead PET Center for
Preventing and Reversing Atherosclerosis,
Memorial Hermann Hospital, University of
Texas Medical School at Houston, Houston,
Texas

AMIR LOTFI, MD, FSCAI
Associate Professor of Medicine, Tufts
University School of Medicine; Division of
Cardiology, Baystate Medical Center, Tufts
University, Springfield, Massachusetts

DONALD R. LYNCH Jr, MD
Fellow, Interventional Cardiology, Division of
Cardiovascular Medicine, Stanford University
Medical Center, Stanford University School of
Medicine, Stanford, California

JAYA MALLIDI, MD, MHS
Interventional Cardiology Fellow, Division of
Cardiology, Baystate Medical Center, Tufts
University, Springfield, Massachusetts

JAMIL MAYET, MD, FESC, FACC
International Centre for Circulatory
Health, National Heart and Lung Institute,
Imperial College London, London,
United Kingdom

JAMES K. MIN, MD
Department of Radiology, Dalio Institute of
Cardiovascular Imaging, New York-
Presbyterian Hospital, Weill Cornell Medical
College, New York, New York

DANYAAL S. MOIN, MD
Division of Cardiovascular Medicine,
Department of Medicine, Stony Brook
University Medical Center, Stony Brook,
New York

SUKHJINDER NIJJER, BSc, MBChB, MRCP
Interventional Cardiology Fellow, International
Centre for Circulatory Health, National Heart
and Lung Institute, Imperial College London,
London, United Kingdom

RICARDO PETRACO, MD, MRCP
Clinical Lecturer, International Centre for
Circulatory Health, National Heart and Lung
Institute, Imperial College London, London,
United Kingdom

HABIB SAMADY, MD, FACC, FSCAI
Director, Interventional Cardiology and
Cardiac Catheterization Laboratory, Emory
University Hospital; Professor of Medicine,
Division of Cardiology, Department of
Medicine, Emory University School of
Medicine, Atlanta, Georgia

SAYAN SEN, BSc, MBBS, MRCP, PhD
Consultant Cardiologist and Clinical
Lecturer, International Centre for Circulatory
Health, National Heart and Lung Institute,
Imperial College London, London, United
Kingdom

**ARNOLD H. SETO, MD, MPA, FSCAI,
FACC**
Assistant Clinical Professor, University of
California, Irvine Medical Center, Orange,
California; Section Chief, Cardiology, Long
Beach Veterans Affairs Medical Center, Long
Beach, California

DAVID TEHRANI, MD, MS
Resident, Medicine, University of Chicago,
Chicago, Illinois; Long Beach Veterans Affairs
Medical Center, Long Beach, California

ALESSANDRO VENEZIANI, PhD
Associate Professor, Department of
Mathematics and Computer Science, Emory
University, Atlanta, Georgia

CONTENTS

History and Development of Coronary Flow Reserve and Fractional Flow Reserve   **397**
for Clinical Applications
Nils P. Johnson, Richard L. Kirkeeide, and K. Lance Gould

> We discuss the historical development of clinical coronary physiology, emphasizing coronary flow reserve (CFR) and fractional flow reserve (FFR). Our analysis focuses on the clinical motivations and technologic advances that prompted and enabled the application of physiology for patient diagnosis. CFR grew from the general concepts of physiologic and coronary reserve, linking the anatomic severity of a lesion to its impact on hyperemic flow. FFR developed from existing models relating pressure measurements to the potential for flow to increase after removing a stenosis. Because pressure measurements have proved easier and more robust than flow measurements, FFR has become the dominant metric.

The Concept of Functional Percutaneous Coronary Intervention: Why Physiologic   **411**
Lesion Assessment Is Integral to Coronary Angiography
Danyaal S. Moin and Allen Jeremias

> The gold standard for assessing the severity of coronary stenoses has been coronary angiography. However, multicenter randomized clinical trials have demonstrated that treatment decisions based on angiography alone do not guarantee benefit to patients. Fractional flow reserve provides physiologic lesion assessment of coronary stenoses. The use of physiology improves clinical outcomes when used for decision making for coronary revascularization. In the era of increased scrutiny of appropriateness of cardiac catheterization and percutaneous coronary intervention, the use of physiologic assessment of the severity of coronary stenoses should be considered an integral adjunct to the anatomic evaluation provided by the coronary angiogram.

Limitations and Pitfalls of Fractional Flow Reserve Measurements and   **419**
Adenosine-Induced Hyperemia
Arnold H. Seto, David Tehrani, and Morton J. Kern

> Coronary hemodynamic measurements provide a critical tool to assess the ischemic potential of coronary stenoses. Fractional flow reserve (FFR) is a reliable method to relate translesional coronary pressures to hyperemic myocardial blood flow. Although a basic understanding in FFR can be quickly achieved, many of the nuances and potential pitfalls require special attention. The authors discuss the practical setup of coronary pressure measurement, the most common pitfalls in technique and ways to avoid them, and the limitations of available pharmacologic hyperemic methods.

Fractional flow reserve (FFR) has become widely used for physiologic assessment of intermediate coronary lesions. The Fractional Flow Reserve to Determine Appropriateness of Angioplasty in Moderate Coronary Stenoses (DEFER) trial established the safety of deferring angioplasty for moderate lesions that are not functionally significant. DEFER and Fractional Flow Reserve versus Angiography for Multivessel Evaluation 1 trials established the feasibility of FFR-guided intervention in stable and unstable patients with moderate coronary lesions, translating to improved clinical outcome and reduced number of unnecessary stents. This article reviews the trials establishing FFR as an important tool for on-the-table functional assessment of coronary lesions.

Although coronary microcirculatory dysfunction occurs in numerous cardiac conditions and influences prognosis, it has been largely ignored in clinical practice due to the lack of adequate methods for its assessment. Microcirculatory dysfuntion may result from a variety of causes, including structural remodelling (arterioles or capillaries), dysregulation (paradoxical arteriolar vasoconstriction), hypersensitivity to vasoactive factors or adrenergic drive, and extravascular compression of collapsable elements. Thus, the selection of a method to interrogate coronary microcirculation should be based on the suspected cause of dysfunction. This article reviews such assessment tools and their prognostic information.

This article assesses the data from contemporary human studies to address some of the common assumptions regarding hyperemic and baseline physiology in the context of the baseline pressure-derived index of instant wave-free ratio and the hyperemic index of fractional flow reserve. The article aims to determine if the available evidence supports the continued investigation, development, and use of baseline indices.

Fractional flow reserve (FFR) is a well-established invasive tool to assess the physiologic significance of a coronary stenosis. Several randomized trials proved the safety of deferring revascularization based on FFR in subjects with stable coronary artery disease with single or multivessel disease. Subjects with tandem or bifurcations lesions, left main disease, and acute coronary syndromes were not included in these trials. Unique hemodynamic changes occur in each of these situations, making the measurement and interpretation of FFR challenging. This article reviews the technical aspects of assessing FFR and literature supporting FFR-guided revascularization in each of these situations.

Fractional flow reserve derived from coronary computed tomography angiography (FFR$_{CT}$) has emerged as a powerful tool for the assessment of flow-limiting coronary stenoses. To date, FFR$_{CT}$ is the only noninvasive imaging modality for the depiction of lesion-specific ischemia and large prospective multicenter studies have established its high diagnostic value. The nature of FFR$_{CT}$ allows the prediction of functional outcome of coronary stenting, which will expand the role of cardiac computed tomography in the evaluation and management of coronary artery disease.

Coronary endothelial function regulation by wall shear stress (WSS), the frictional force of blood exerted against the vessel wall, can help explain the focal propensity of plaque development in an environment of systemic atherosclerosis risk factors. Sustained abnormal pathologic WSS leads to a proatherogenic endothelial cell phenotype, plaque progression and transformation, and adaptive vascular remodeling in site-specific areas. Assessing dynamic coronary plaque compositional changes in vivo remains challenging; however, recent advances in intravascular image acquisition and processing may provide swifter WSS calculations and make possible larger prospective investigations on the prognostic value of WSS in patients with coronary atherosclerosis.

INTRAVASCULAR PHYSIOLOGY

ISSUE OF RELATED INTEREST

Cardiology Clinics, February 2015 (Vol. 33, No. 1)
Vascular Disease
Leonardo Clavijo, *Editor*
Available at: http://www.cardiology.theclinics.com/

THE CLINICS ARE NOW AVAILABLE ONLINE!

Access your subscription at:
www.theclinics.com

PREFACE

Coronary Physiology: Basic Concepts and Clinical Applications

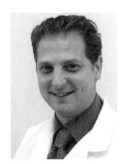

Allen Jeremias, MD, MSc
Editor

The routine clinical application of coronary physiology has become available with the introduction of Fractional Flow Reserve (FFR) over 20 years ago. The premise of FFR is to assess the hemodynamic significance of a coronary stenosis by comparing distal coronary pressure to the aortic pressure as a surrogate for coronary flow. Since the original description by Pijls and colleagues in 1993, more than 1500 articles have been published containing the keyword "FFR", and coronary pressure measurements have become mainstream. Nevertheless, despite convincing clinical trial evidence demonstrating the benefits of FFR, clinical adoption remains low with only about 10% of coronary angiograms undergoing an FFR evaluation.

This issue of *Interventional Cardiology Clinics* is dedicated to coronary physiology, providing an excellent overview of the basic concepts, historical advances in the field, clinical trial evidence, practical applications, and future developments. The authors are international experts in coronary physiology and have significantly contributed to the scientific progress in this space. In addition to an in-depth discussion on FFR (including its limitations and pitfalls), there is a focus on Coronary Flow Reserve in the context of assessing microvascular disease, the association of wall shear stress and plaque progression, the potential advantages of using resting pressure indices such as instant wave-free ratio, and the noninvasive evaluation of FFR derived from coronary computed tomography angiography. It is my hope that this issue will contribute to the much needed expansion of physiology measurements in routine clinical practice in an era of increasing scrutiny of coronary revascularization procedures.

I would like to extend my gratitude to all authors who contributed to this issue of *Interventional Cardiology Clinics*. I hope that this issue provides a relevant and up-to-date overview of coronary physiology and will help implement some of these concepts into daily clinical practice.

Allen Jeremias, MD, MSc
Department of Medicine
Division of Cardiovascular Medicine
Health Sciences Center, T16-080
Stony Brook, NY 11794-8160, USA
E-mail address:
allen.jeremias@stonybrookmedicine.edu

Intervent Cardiol Clin 4 (2015) ix
http://dx.doi.org/10.1016/j.iccl.2015.08.001
2211-7458/15/$ – see front matter © 2015 Published by Elsevier Inc.

History and Development of Coronary Flow Reserve and Fractional Flow Reserve for Clinical Applications

Nils P. Johnson, MD, MS*, Richard L. Kirkeeide, PhD,
K. Lance Gould, MD

KEYWORDS

- Clinical coronary physiology • Coronary flow reserve • Fractional flow reserve
- Historical development

KEY POINTS

- Clinical coronary physiology developed as an applied branch of pure physiology with a specific goal of diagnosing and treating patients with coronary artery disease.
- The historical development of clinical coronary physiology can be understood though a focus on both clinical motivations and technologic advances.
- Revascularization risk and angiographic ambiguity motivated the development of clinical coronary physiology, whereas the development of flow and pressure sensors made it a reality.
- Coronary flow reserve (CFR) equals the ratio of flow between hyperemia and resting conditions and first linked anatomic severity to physiologic reserve.
- Fractional flow reserve (FFR) equals the ratio of maximum flow between the stenotic artery and the same artery free from stenosis and, under certain conditions, can be measured before intervention with pressure sensors.

INTRODUCTION

In this review we discuss the history and development of clinical, invasive coronary physiology. By emphasizing the word *clinical*, we draw an immediate distinction between medicine (an applied field whose goal is patient care) and pure physiology (a branch of science devoted to understanding the functional mechanisms of life). Like engineering from physics, clinical medicine borrows from physiology but with the distinct purpose of practical intervention instead of rigorous description. Unlike a controlled animal model, humans typically display a host of simultaneous variations that we cannot quantify

perfectly. Nevertheless, such patients appear in our clinics, emergency departments, and hospital wards requiring diagnosis and treatment. Therefore, *clinical* physiology sacrifices purity for pragmatism – summarized by the quotation, "all models are wrong, but some are useful."[1]

Our review begins with the motivating forces behind clinical coronary physiology. Next we detail the evolution of technical developments, both pharmacologic and sensors. Finally, we place the conceptual development of CFR and FFR in a historical context, linked to clinical motivations and technical developments. We focus on CFR and FFR because these 2 metrics have the longest history and broadest application. As summarized in

---

Financial Support and Relationships with Industry: see last page of the article.
Division of Cardiology, Department of Medicine, Weatherhead PET Center for Preventing and Reversing Atherosclerosis, Memorial Hermann Hospital, University of Texas Medical School at Houston, 6431 Fannin Street, Room MSB 4.256, Houston, TX 77030, USA
* Corresponding author.
E-mail address: Nils.Johnson@uth.tmc.edu

Intervent Cardiol Clin 4 (2015) 397–410
http://dx.doi.org/10.1016/j.iccl.2015.06.001
2211-7458/15/$ – see front matter © 2015 Elsevier Inc. All rights reserved.

Table 1, a large number of invasive metrics has been proposed for studying coronary physiology. CFR and FFR stand apart, however, for their longevity and depth of study. As stated presciently in 1997, "The preference for one physiologic technique may come from advances in guide wire capabilities and handling characteristics, ease of signal interpretation and integration into the specific catheterization laboratory system."[2]

CLINICAL MOTIVATIONS

Two clinical forces have spurred development of clinical coronary physiology: risk of revascularization and angiographic ambiguity. Excerpts from a 1997 article[2] capture these elements:

- Procedural risk: "... in so performing [percutaneous transluminal coronary angioplasty], a previously stable (and functionally not significant) lesion might be activated and a deleterious 'restenosis' process triggered. In fact, it is expected that in 20% to 30% of such patients, a clinically relevant restenosis will occur within 6 months. It is therefore unclear whether the risk of dilating a functionally

Table 1
Proposed indexes for invasive coronary physiology

Index	Full Name	Year	Developer(s)	Reference	Publications[a]
CFR (or CFVR)	Coronary flow (velocity) reserve	1974	Gould	53	>2000
ΔP	Translesion pressure gradient	1979[b]	Grüntzig	4	N/A[c]
Pd/Pa	Various terms, usually simply Pd/Pa	1985[b]	Wijns	73	
IHDVPS	Instant, hyperemic, diastolic velocity/pressure slope	1989	Mancini	74	<10
FFR	Fractional flow reserve	1993	Pijls and De Bruyne	63	>1000
d-FFR	Diastolic FFR	2000	Abe	75	<10
HMR	Hyperemic microvascular resistance	2001	AMC[d]	76	≈50
HSR (and BSR)	Hyperemic (and basal) stenosis resistance	2002 (and 2012)		77	≈10
PFLA	Pressure-flow loop area	2002	Ovadia-Blechman	78	<10
PTC	Pulse transmission coefficient	2002	Lerman	79	<10
IMR	Index of microcirculatory resistance	2003	Fearon	80	≈50
DCVR	Diastolic coronary vasodilator reserve	2004	Serruys	81	<10
dp_{v50}	Translesion gradient at 50 cm/s	2006	Marques	82	<10
CDP (or LFC)	Pressure drop (or lesion flow) coefficient (equivalent to the Euler number)	2007	Banerjee	83	≈20
iFR	Instantaneous wave-free ratio	2012	Davies	84	≈20

Abbreviations: Pa, aortic pressure; Pd, distal coronary pressure.
[a] Approximate PubMed search on full or related name in title or abstract or Scopus search for citations of primary reference.
[b] Refers to its clinical application in humans, as the index had been proposed previously.
[c] These measures have become so common that specific publication counts are not applicable.
[d] Academic Medical Center in Amsterdam, Netherlands, including Meuwissen, Piek, Siebes, Spaan, and van de Hoef.
Data from Refs.[4,53,63,73–84]

nonsignificant but angiographically intermediate stenosis outweighs the risk of leaving such a lesion untreated."

- Angiographic ambiguity: "It has been shown that in a randomly selected group of asymptomatic 60-year old men, the prevalence of apparently significant coronary stenoses is 20%. Therefore, one must assume that in a number of such patients, the presence of a lesion may be coincidental and that a direct relation between the angiographic lesion and the chest pain is unclear."

Each of these motivations will now be discussed in further detail. The first motivation (procedural risk) has diminished during the past decades whereas the second motivation (angiographic ambiguity) has, if anything, intensified.

Risk of Revascularization

The procedure-related risk of revascularization must not exceed its potential benefit. As with all treatments in medicine, the balance between these 2 forces represents a dynamic process. Technical advances reduce therapeutic risk, whereas optimization of patient selection maximizes clinical advantages. Because a major motivation for clinical coronary physiology has been to optimize patient selection for revascularization, an understanding of the magnitude of its risk during the developmental period of CFR and FFR remains essential. Although a broad topic, we seek to briefly summarize the trends in risk from coronary artery bypass grafting (CABG) and percutaneous coronary intervention (PCI).

Coronary revascularization via CABG has been performed for more than 50 years, and readers should look elsewhere for a detailed review. Major adverse cardiovascular events from CABG can include death, nonfatal myocardial infarction (MI), and stroke. A meta-analysis of CABG reports between 1990 and 2001 showed an average incidence of 1.7% for in-hospital death, 2.4% for nonfatal MI, and 1.3% for stroke.[3]

As for PCI treatment, the risks of emergent CABG, MI, future vessel closure or stent thrombosis, and subsequent restenosis have decreased since the initial series of balloon angioplasty published in 1979.[4] Although the first publication reported that 14% of patients required urgent or emergent CABG, modern rates have fallen to 0.4%.[5] Likely, this temporal reduction in rates of PCI-induced CABG relates to a combination of clinical experience, patient selection, lesion selection (including application

of FFR, demonstrating an interplay between diagnostic tool and treatment risk), modern antithrombotic medications, and the development of coronary stents.

Procedure-related MI occurs during PCI by a variety of mechanisms, including direct vessel injury, side branch compromise, thrombus formation, and distal embolization. Although the definition and prognostic implications of these infarcts remain debated,[6] their incidence has decreased over the past 35 years. The first balloon angioplasty report in 1979[4] noted that 5% to 10% of patients had a procedure-related MI, whereas a recent randomized trial published in 2010[7] found a rate of less than 1%.

Abrupt vessel closure after balloon angioplasty or stent thrombosis after implantation typically produces a dramatic clinical presentation of acute MI or sudden death. Abrupt vessel closure after balloon angioplasty occurred in approximately 8% of cases,[8] and very early experiences with stents showed a 16% subacute closure rate.[9] But development of dual antiplatelet therapy and refinement of scaffold design and implantation techniques have reduced its frequency to 0.4% over 30 months.[10]

A similar temporal trend also exists for restenosis. After the first series of coronary stent implantation described in 1987,[11] clinical trials by 1994[12,13] had demonstrated improvements, although restenosis remained significant either with balloon dilation or stenting (32% vs 22% in Benestent study at 7 months; 42% vs 32% in STRESS at 6 months). Modern technology has reduced restenosis further by 5- to 10-fold, as demonstrated by a 2010 trial,[7] with 3% to 4% target-lesion and 5% target-vessel revascularization at 12 months using everolimus or zotarolimus drug-eluting stents.

Therefore, the motivation behind clinical coronary physiology driven by revascularization procedural risk has diminished over time. Nevertheless, in the early 1970s when CFR was being developed, only CABG existed. In the early 1990s when FFR was being developed, the risk of emergent PCI-induced CABG was approximately 2% to 4%[5] and the risk of PCI-induced restenosis was approximately 25% at 6 months.[12,13] These high levels of procedure-related risk prompted clinicians to select appropriate patients, such that benefits would be larger.

Angiographic Ambiguity

How can we be sure that an angiographic lesion explains a patient's symptoms or presentation? Is the observed coronary artery disease causal or incidental? If multiple focal lesions exist, which one (or ones) is the culprit? Does the coexisting diffuse coronary atherosclerosis overwhelm the contribution of focal disease? These clinical questions arise frequently from the angiogram, and anatomy alone often fails to provide comprehensive answers.

Autopsy findings of atherosclerosis among people (not patients) who died of other causes provide an estimate of the prevalence of significant, subclinical coronary artery disease. A series of 3832 members of the United States military who died of combat or unintentional injuries between 2001 and 2011 found a ≥50% diameter stenosis in 2.3%, despite an average age of approximately 26 years.[14] Perhaps due to a reduction in risk factors, this prevalence rate is lower than similar autopsy series from the Vietnam (5%) and Korean (15%) wars.[14]

Invasive angiography has probably never been performed as a screening test in a large, asymptomatic, general population, because invasive procedures require some deviation from normal (symptoms, abnormal noninvasive test, or enrichment of risk factors). Large registries of patients with minimal symptoms undergoing invasive angiography, however, allow for an upper bound. The Coronary Artery Surgery Study registry from 1981 analyzed invasive angiograms from 15 sites.[15] A total of 1282 men and 1397 women had nonspecific chest pain and, of this subgroup, 14% of men and 6% of women had either a ≥50% diameter stenosis of the left main or at least 1 ≥70% diameter stenosis elsewhere.

In addition, coronary angiography using CT imaging has been performed in 2 major, multicenter studies of asymptomatic patients published recently. A registry from 12 centers in 6 countries performed noninvasive angiography in 3217 asymptomatic patients without known coronary disease.[16] A total of 546 patients (17%) had a ≥50% diameter stenosis, of which 79 patients (2% of the total) had triple-vessel or left main disease. A randomized trial from 45 sites of 900 asymptomatic diabetes performed noninvasive angiography in 336 patients.[17] A total of 21 patients (6%) had a ≥70% diameter stenosis in a proximal vessel.

Together, these anatomic studies demonstrate a significant burden of subclinical coronary atherosclerosis whose frequency increases with classic risk factors. Therefore, performing coronary angiography on an unselected person (not patient) occasionally uncovers intermediate or severe anatomic disease. For that reason, causality between an angiographic lesion and any clinical complaints or abnormal test result can remain uncertain, particularly in the broad range of so-called intermediate stenoses. The existence of multivessel and diffuse disease only adds a layer of uncertainty.

Therefore, the motivation behind clinical coronary physiology driven by angiographic ambiguity has, if anything, intensified as a result of more available noninvasive anatomic imaging. We face today the same quandary as the clinicians at the beginning of invasive coronary angiography and treatment – namely, how should we determine which lesion (or lesions) to revascularize and which can be deferred for medical therapy alone?

TECHNICAL DEVELOPMENTS

Two types of technical developments have occurred that paved the way for coronary physiology to become a clinical tool. As detailed next, physicians required both potent, clinical, short-acting hyperemic stimuli and robust, miniature flow and pressure sensors. Together these new developments permitted addressing the clinical challenges of procedural risk and angiographic ambiguity (discussed previously).

Clinical Vasodilators

Because coronary autoregulation maintains myocardial blood flow at a reasonably stable level over a wide range of perfusion pressures, resting measurements alone provide limited sensitivity for stenosis severity. Additionally, many patient symptoms occur with activity; therefore, resting conditions do not provide a reasonable surrogate. For these reasons, potent and short-acting vasodilator drugs were necessary for reliable and repeated hyperemic measurements to optimize lesion assessment.

The first techniques for provoking hyperemia were transient coronary occlusions and intracoronary contrast medium injections. Intact patients cannot undergo diagnostic coronary occlusions, and early contrast agents, like Hypaque (a solution of sodium diatrizoate, often 50% or 75%), could provoke reactions like emesis, transient heart block, and ventricular fibrillation. Accordingly, these techniques found their best application in animal models, although temporary coronary occlusion was used during CABG to measure flow reserve[18] and modern contrast agents retain some hyperemic potential.[19]

Dipyridamole was first reported for vasodilator stress imaging in 1978,[20] but its 4-minute infusion followed by a further 4-minute wait for peak effect made it a long-acting tool less suited for invasive measurements. In 1986, papaverine was developed for human intracoronary use[21] followed by intravenous adenosine in 1990,[22] although animal work on both drugs dates back much further by several decades. These medications produced more potent hyperemia than contrast agents,[23] with generally fewer side effects, although papaverine can induce QT prolongation and polymorphic ventricular fibrillation.[24] Additionally their onset of action is rapid, approximately 5 to 10 seconds for intracoronary adenosine, 30 to 60 seconds for intracoronary papaverine, and 60 to 120 seconds for intravenous adenosine.[25]

Several additional drugs have since been introduced to augment flow for invasive measurements in humans: ATP in 2003,[26] nitroprusside in 2004,[27] nicorandil in 2006,[28] and regadenoson in 2011.[29] Together these newer agents, along with older tools of contrast medium, papaverine and adenosine, provide trade-offs among hyperemic potency, duration of action, cost, side-effect profile, and regulatory availability. Their development was essential, however, to the clinical uptake of CFR and FFR as routine diagnostic tools.

Flow and Pressure Measurements

Intracardiac and intracoronary flow and pressure measurements have a long history. Donald Gregg devoted 2 chapters of his classic 1950 book, *Coronary Circulation in Health and Disease*, to "Experimental Approaches to the Coronary Circulation. Coronary Flow. Its Determination" and "Experimental Approaches to the Coronary Circulation. Preparations. Cardiac Pressures and their Determinations."[30] A review article from 1987[31] discussed the strengths and limitations of invasive techniques, such as coronary sinus thermodilution, video densitometry, and Doppler flow probes. Notably, our progressive methods to measure flow and pressure track our ability to understand the physiology, make clinical diagnoses, and evaluate therapeutic interventions.

Flow Sensor Development

Advances in miniaturization led to the 1963 description of an electromagnetic flow meter that could be implanted in animals.[32] By the late 1960s and early 1970s, such devices could be obtained commercially and led to a great interest and exploration of intact physiology in a variety of animals.

For instantaneous measurements of flow in intact humans, however, the first work in 1971[33] and then in 1977[34] used a Doppler probe mounted at the tip of coronary catheter, permitting recordings only at the ostium. Later, an epicardial suction cup was developed in 1981[35] that permitted distal coronary flow measurements during bypass surgery.[18] An intracoronary 3F Doppler sensor introduced in 1985 extended recordings to both intact humans (not just during bypass surgery) and distal coronary branches (not only the ostium).[36] The technology was further refined to 0.018-inch Doppler wires by 1992,[37,38] and modern 0.014-inch Doppler wires by 1996.[39]

Separate from Doppler technology, intracoronary thermal methods have also been used to measure flow. Bolus thermodilution techniques introduced in 2001 took advantage of the temperature sensitivity of standard, intracoronary pressure wires to yield the transit time, an inverse surrogate for flow.[40,41] Continuous coronary thermodilution proposed in 2007 required a proximal infusion system but measured volumetric flow rates (mL/min).[42] Most recently, thermal anemometry was suggested as an alternative in 2013.[43] Of these techniques, only bolus thermodilution can be obtained routinely on a commercial basis.

Pressure Sensor Development

Initially Grüntzig and colleagues[4] used large, fluid-filled catheters for angioplasty cases. Later work reduced the size to 2F,[44] but even so these larger catheters could artificially impede flow: "the pressure gradient across the stenosis provides only an index of the severity of the lesion since the insertion of the dilatation catheter … contributes to the stenosis."[4]

By 1991, however, an 0.018-inch fiber optic wire had been developed[45] followed by an 0.015-inch fluid-filled wire in 1993[46] and then an 0.014-inch piezoelectric sensor a few years later.[47] The stenosis induced by an 0.015-inch wire is negligible except for critical lesions whose severity rarely remains uncertain at angiography.[46] Modern FFR pressure sensors are mainly standard 0.014-inch diameter, although a rapid exchange 0.022-inch catheter has been introduced recently.[48] Manufacturers differ between piezoelectric and fiber optic sensors, in addition to overall wire performance and handling.

CORONARY FLOW RESERVE

Concept

The general concept of physiologic reserve has been applied to many organs. For example, other investigators have proposed *renal reserve* for augmented kidney function after ingestion of protein or amino acids[49] and *cerebral reserve* for cerebral blood flow increases in response to acetazolamide provocation.[50] The joint term, coronary reserve can be found in PubMed as far back as April 1963,[51] although that date likely reflects the specific search engine as opposed to the actual literature. The concept, if not the term, can be found much earlier; for example, Gregg wrote in 1950, "the inability of the heart to increase or even maintain its blood supply in the presence of an augmented load indicates an almost complete lack of reserve."[30]

The senior author of this article (KLG) was influenced both by Gregg's pioneering work and the contemporary developments from Germany, especially Michael Tauchert.[52] As a representative example of his work from early 1973, Fig. 1 shows myocardial perfusion (measured using the argon technique) at rest and after dipyridamole infusion in a patient with an ischemic cardiomyopathy.[52] Its English abstract used the term, coronary vascular reserve, as the ratio of hyperemic to baseline coronary vascular resistance, essentially adjusting CFR for the aortic driving pressures.

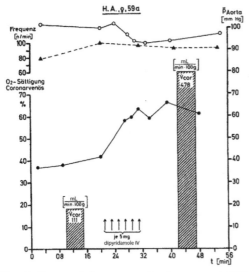

Fig. 1. German influence on development of CFR. Patient H.A., a 59-year-old woman with a clinical diagnosis of ischemic cardiomyopathy, underwent measurement of coronary blood flow using the argon technique both at rest (1.11 mL/min/g) and after intravenous dipyridamole infusion (4.78 mL/min/g). Solid dots represent coronary venous oxygen saturation (O₂-Sättigung Coronarvenös), triangles document heart rate (Frequenz [n/min]), and open circles denote mean aortic pressure ($\bar{p}_{Aorta}$ [mm Hg]). IV, intravenous; Vcor, coronary flow. (From Tauchert M. Coronary reserve capacity and maximum oxygen consumption of the human heart. Basic Res Cardiol 1973;68:196. [in German]; with permission.)

Initial Article

The senior author (KLG) of this review first published the specific phrase "coronary flow reserve" in January 1974,[53] although similar notions of "coronary reserve" or "coronary vascular reserve" existed, as discussed previously. Its intuition derived from Fig. 2, which compared hyperemic responses after intracoronary contrast injections in instrumented dogs with electromagnetic flow meters on a variably stenotic left circumflex artery. For mild stenoses (approximately <50% diameter), flow increased by approximately 4-fold with hyperemia; but for severe stenoses (approximately 70%–90% diameter), flow increased by less than 2-fold.

Why did the specific concept of CFR from early 1974 gain traction whereas previous presentations of similar ideas did not? Although other groups were mainly focused on understanding "pure" coronary physiology, the senior author (KLG) differentiated his research by applying coronary physiology to anatomic stenosis. Relating CFR to epicardial stenosis, as in the right-hand plot of Fig. 2, easily linked clinical questions to physiologic explanations: Why does a patient with a discrete 50% diameter stenosis not have symptoms? And why does a patient with a 70% stenosis only have exertional but not resting symptoms? Now these questions were answered, because flow can still increase approximately 4-fold at 50% stenosis while resting flow remains preserved well past a 70% stenosis. Also, beyond explanation, the initial CFR article hinted at the possibility of guiding treatment: "possibly a hyperemic/base-line flow ratio of less than 1.5 would be an indication for [coronary artery bypass] surgery."[53]

Previous presentations either discussed the issue generally or did not link CFR to anatomic severity. For example, Gregg wrote in 1950, "when a coronary artery is only moderately constricted, the flow is only temporarily reduced ... unless the degree of constriction is extreme. Presumably, this compensatory vasodilation exists in man and operates to avoid the untoward effects of temporary ischemia which may appear during exercise"[30] but did not quantitatively relate the "degree of constriction" to restricted flow. Similarly, Tauchert in 1973[52] listed CFR for 25 patients with a mean value of 4.60 ± 0.27 but did not relate it to their angiographic findings.

Evolution of Coronary Flow Reserve

CFR evolved in 3 separate yet related directions after its 1974 introduction. First, invasive

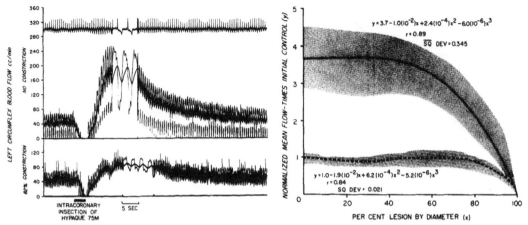

Fig. 2. Concept behind CFR. As noted in the animal model that introduced CFR in 1974,[53] the flow increase after a hyperemic stimulus (here an intracoronary injection of Hypaque 75M contrast medium) diminishes with progressive epicardial stenosis. The left panel shows 2 typical phasic flow tracings made in the left circumflex with a 0% diameter stenosis ("no constriction" [*top*]) and an 82% diameter stenosis (*bottom*). The right panel aggregates the data from 12 dogs, where the shaded area represents the individual scatter about the group trend line (third-order polynomial fit). r, correlation coefficient; SQ DEV, mean square of deviations. (*From* Gould KL, Lipscomb K, Hamilton GW. Physiologic basis for assessing critical coronary stenosis. Instantaneous flow response and regional distribution during coronary hyperemia as measures of coronary flow reserve. Am J Cardiol 1974;33:87–94; with permission.)

measurements expanded in humans with improved flow sensors (as previously discussed). After initial exploration of CFR in a variety of clinical scenarios through 1998,[54] CFR was studied in the DEBATE trials in 1997 and 2000 as a guide for provisional instead of routine stent implantation.[55,56] Ultimately, routine stent implantation became so effective and inexpensive that any added value from therapeutic CFR measurement was eroded. The rise of FFR in the mid-1990s served to diminish further the enthusiasm for CFR, because pressure could be measured more robustly than flow. Despite a new wave of physiology metrics that incorporated flow, as detailed in Table 1, invasive CFR has been chosen as the basis for an ongoing, outcomes-based clinical trial,[57] reflecting its vast literature and strong physiologic basis.

Second, anatomic modeling of CFR from the angiogram gave rise to the related concept of stenosis flow reserve in 1986 during the development and adoption of invasive, quantitative coronary angiography.[58] Although predicting physiology from anatomy suffers from fundamental limitations due to biologic variability and imperfect image resolution, stenosis flow reserve models of CFR served as the intellectual predecessor to current simulations, like modeling of FFR from CT angiography and related techniques.[59]

Third, CFR launched the field of noninvasive perfusion imaging, where it is sometimes called myocardial perfusion reserve to distinguish epicardial from myocardial flow. As noted in the initial 1974 article, "flow distribution may be evaluated in man with the gamma camera … A more physiologic approach might be utilized if responses … were established for normal and diseased human coronary arteries by clinical studies using a … gamma camera."[53] The last 2 figures of the 1974 article display perfusion data after tracer injection at rest and during hyperemia. Now, 40 years later, a vast literature exists of noninvasive CFR measurements in approximately 15,000 patients or subjects from more than 250 publications.[60] Currently CFR can be measured noninvasively using cardiac positron emission tomography, MRI, CT, and myocardial contrast or Doppler echocardiography.

FRACTIONAL FLOW RESERVE
Concept
Conceptually FFR makes a prediction about the future, as depicted in Fig. 3. FFR involves a before/after comparison of maximum flow between the current, stenotic artery, and a potential future artery free from stenosis. Making direct hyperemic flow measurements before and after removing the stenosis requires revascularization, itself the very clinical question being posed. Therefore, the key concept behind FFR states that – under certain conditions and assumptions – a hyperemic pressure measurement before revascularization can provide the same information.

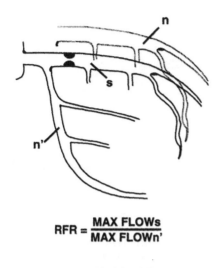

$$RFR = \frac{MAX\ FLOWs}{MAX\ FLOWn'}$$

$$FFR = \frac{MAX\ FLOWs}{MAX\ FLOWn}$$

In case of ISOLATED coronary artery stenosis

RFR = FFR

(per unit of tissue mass)

Fig. 3. Concept behind FFR. As depicted in the first human study of FFR from 1994,[67] FFR equals the ratio of maximal flow in a stenotic artery (s) to the same artery without the stenosis (n'). Relative CFR (RFR) equals the ratio of maximum flow in the stenotic artery to a neighboring, normal artery (n). For isolated coronary artery stenosis, RFR equals FFR when normalized for distal myocardial mass. (*From* De Bruyne B, Baudhuin T, Melin JA, et al. Coronary flow reserve calculated from pressure measurements in humans. Validation with positron emission tomography. Circulation 1994;89:1013–22; with permission.)

Previous Work

Even before the FFR model was proposed in 1993, it had been appreciated that the relative distal pressure could provide the ratio of maximum flow in a stenotic artery to maximum flow without the stenosis. A 1977 article from the Iowa group led by Donald Young (and including the author, RLK, as a young graduate student) proposed a schematic model of a general circulation,[61] shown in Fig. 4. Their derivation began by noting, "a useful index for characterizing the effect of a stenosis is the ratio of the maximum flow rate in the presence of the stenosis ... to the maximum flow rate without the stenosis ... This ratio represents the reduction in the vascular bed reserve due to a stenotic obstruction. For the simple model...the maximum flow rate is given by the equation ...", and went on to derive the ratio of distal perfusion pressure to driving aortic pressure, calling it the "vascular bed reserve ratio." Their experimental work created femoral and carotid stenoses in dogs, but did not explore the coronary circulation specifically.

Later dog work in 1990 from the 2 senior authors of this article (RLK and KLG) applied the same conceptual framework to the coronary circulation during a study of relative CFR.[62] In that discussion, we noted that "relative coronary flow reserve reflects more specifically the effects of the stenosis independent of and not affected by the other physiologic variables ... Relative flow reserve more accurately defines physiologic stenosis severity because it is not affected by variability in pressure or heart rate within the same patient or among patients ... Relative

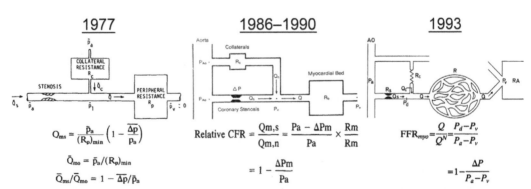

Fig. 4. Historical development of fractional flow reserve. Over a 16-year period, several groups proposed similar models that used pressure-only equations to derive the ratio of maximal flow with a stenosis to maximal flow without a stenosis. On the left, work by Young and colleagues[61] in 1977 proposed a conceptual model for a generalized arterial supply and peripheral bed. In the center, work by Gould and colleagues[72] in 1986 applied a similar model to the coronary circulation. On the right, work by Pijls and colleagues[63] in 1993 extended the model with a rigorous concept of collateral flow. (*From* Refs.[61,63,72])

coronary flow reserve is altered only by stenosis severity." Then we proceeded to "[provide] … the following readily derived simple equations relating flow reserve to pressure and distal bed resistance" and went on to demonstrate that relative CFR equals the ratio of distal coronary pressure to aortic driving pressure, as shown in Fig. 4.

As made clear by the discussion from 1990,[62] relative CFR or FFR focuses attention on the epicardial stenosis. Because of defined therapies for epicardial lesions, namely PCI and CABG, such a focus naturally links diagnosis with treatment. By contrast, absolute CFR incorporates both epicardial and microvascular contributions plus systemic hemodynamics. We lamented previously that "most invasive or noninvasive clinical methods as now used provide measurements of either absolute or relative coronary flow reserve, but not both,"[62] reflecting the situation in the late 1980s. An ongoing study,[57] however, combining CFR and FFR will determine if an important diagnostic or therapeutic role exists based on their simultaneous assessment.

Initial Article

The foundation article for FFR in 1993[63] brought together all the stands, discussed previously, in its development – substantial risk from PCI itself, angiographic ambiguity, clinical hyperemic drugs, miniature pressure sensors, and a theoretic framework for interpreting the ratio of distal coronary to driving aortic pressure. As clarified early in that first FFR article, "there are three reasons why pressure measurements have not been useful for assessment of flow":

- "First, the instrument used for pressure measurement in previous studies (in most cases, the balloon catheter) is unsuitable because its size is too large compared with the size of the coronary artery."
- "Second, most previous measurements have been made in the basal state … Although the necessity of maximum vasodilation generally is recognized at present, it has not been applied to measurements of pressure gradients in a number of previous studies."
- "Third, in previous studies for assessing stenosis severity by pressure measurements, coronary flow … has been related to transstenotic pressure gradient … this approach is fundamentally limited because it fails to recognize that the stenosis is only one part of a complex hydrodynamic system of which other parts

may also affect the influence of the stenosis on blood flow."

To address the third point, a key added component for the FFR model[63] compared with prior work[61,62] was a rigorous explanation for the collateral circulation. As such, the model could distinguish between contributions from the epicardial conduit (termed, *fractional coronary artery flow reserve* [FFR_{cor}]) and from collateral channels (termed, *fractional collateral blood flow* in a 1995 article[64]) to net myocardial blood flow (termed, *FFR of the myocardium* [FFR_{myo}]). This point is made explicit in the 1993 discussion, noting that "coronary FFR should be calculated using … rather than … as initially proposed by Gould … but incomplete in failing to account for collateral flow."

Evolution of Fractional Flow Reserve

Impressively, the FFR model from 1993 has not required any major conceptual changes. Perhaps because FFR itself evolved from prior work dating back to 1977 (previously discussed) the original presentation has withstood the test of time. Several refinements have occurred to its framework, including accounting for serial lesions[65] and diffuse disease[66] using pull-back techniques. Already in 1993 the contribution of venous pressure was appreciated as negligible for myocardial FFR: "If venous pressure is not elevated … the venous pressure may be neglected because its influence … is minimal in that case."[63] Most of the FFR evolution during the past 2 decades has been practical (better wires and pressure sensors, expanded options for pharmacologic hyperemia, and more user-friendly acquisition systems) or clinical (correlations with noninvasive stress tests, observational outcomes data, and randomized controlled trials).

SUMMARY
Coronary Physiology—Bench to Bedside

If no man is an island, then no idea develops outside of its historical context. This framework of understanding holds particularly true for clinical coronary physiology – the application of physiologic principles for the clinical diagnosis and treatment of coronary artery disease. Without sensors and medications to make routine, intracoronary measurements of pressure and flow in intact humans, clinical coronary physiology could not exist. As previously discussed, the interplay between the clinical motivations of revascularization risk and angiographic ambiguity and the technical developments of hyperemic stimuli and pressure or flow sensors enabled – and to some extent probably even propelled – the conceptual frameworks behind CFR and FFR.

Both initial articles for CFR in 1974[53] and FFR in 1993[63] used animal models, but human translation began soon afterward. Three years later in 1977, 58 patients had undergone intracoronary CFR measurement using a Doppler sensor and contrast medium hyperemia.[34] FFR published its first series of 22 patients the next year, in 1994.[67] Currently the size of the FFR market is estimated at approximately 250,000 procedures per year (Mona Tirén, St Jude Medical, personal communication, 2014) and more than 1 million patients total have undergone its measurement – a canonical example of bench to bedside translation from the 5 dogs studied in 1993.

Fundamentally we can only measure intracoronary pressure and flow. Metrics such as resistance represent abstract and derived quantities. Perhaps in the future combined measurements will advance clinical care further[57] because, as summarized elegantly in 1997, "pressure and flow represent the two sides of the same coin ... from the physiologic point of view, both techniques are highly complementary."[2]

Lessons from the Past Applied to the Present

In the early 1970s, invasive coronary angiograms and surgical bypass were dominant, mainstream themes both in the literature and in daily practice. The early articles and investigators (previously discussed) were remote, hidden in the physiology or German literature, unrecognized outliers, and without clinical relevance to cardiology. At that time, however, to the senior author, a glaringly obvious signal arose from this diverse literature that powerfully related to percent diameter stenosis on the coronary angiogram – reactive or contrast-induced hyperemia, fluid dynamic equations, and pharmacologic stress perfusion imaging. To the senior author, the signals in the literature were so strong, so obvious, and even overwhelming that he found an obsession with integrating, understanding, and developing the experimental surgery required to acquire definitive data, answers, and thence technology for clinically measuring absolute myocardial perfusion and CFR.

This brief recounting of cardiovascular thinking mirrors nearly exactly a current clinical issue. Despite the technological and clinical advances previously outlined, a major question remains in cardiology without established explanation or potential solution: Why do randomized revascularization trials of stable patients fail to reduce MI or mortality significantly? One explanation is that these procedures, even when physiologically guided, do not alter the natural history of the disease while relieving symptoms. In that case, the commonest justification for revascularization given to patients "to prevent a heart attack or death"[68] is misleading inducement. When fully informed, a third of patients elected against the recommended procedure.[69] How does the profession resolve this issue – is there a potential positive answer, or only that we need to advise our patients more truthfully?

The current central issue in cardiology parallels the prior evolution of clinical coronary pathophysiology. The authors see a glaring signal from current, diverse literature that most likely explains why randomized revascularization trials do not reduce MI or death. A new explicit physiologic synthesis hypothesizes an answer to this issue. It also suggests a potential physiologic solution for proving revascularization reduces MI and death in appropriately selected patients or definitively showing that it does not. This historical review is not appropriate for publishing that synthesis. Two recent editorials[70,71] and their references, however, contain some of its elements. The authors challenge the readers to consider those oblique published views as historical parallels to this central issue in invasive cardiology or other new concepts in cardiovascular medicine. Those unaware of history may be doomed to repeat it. Those aware and open to its lessons can make history a springboard into the future, proving the aphorism that there is nothing new under the sun.

FINANCIAL SUPPORT AND RELATIONSHIPS WITH INDUSTRY

All authors received internal funding from the Weatherhead PET Center for Preventing and Reversing Atherosclerosis and have signed nonfinancial, nondisclosure agreements with St Jude Medical and Volcano Corporation to discuss coronary physiology projects.

N.P. Johnson has received significant institutional research support from St. Jude Medical (for CONTRAST, NCT02184117) and Volcano Corporation (for DEFINE-FLOW, NCT02328820).

R.L. Kirkeeide has no further disclosures.

K. L. Gould is the 510 (k) applicant for cfrQuant, a software package for quantifying absolute flow using cardiac positron emission tomography. All royalties go to a University of

Texas scholarship fund. The University of Texas has a commercial, nonexclusive agreement with Positron Corporation to distribute and market cfrQuant in exchange for royalties. K.L. Gould retains the ability, however, to distribute cost-free versions to selected collaborators for research.

REFERENCES

1. George E. P. Box quotes. Available at: http://en.wikiquote.org/wiki/George_E._P._Box. Accessed January 12, 2015.

2. Kern MJ, de Bruyne B, Pijls NH. From research to clinical practice: current role of intracoronary physiologically based decision making in the cardiac catheterization laboratory. J Am Coll Cardiol 1997;30:613–20.

3. Nalysnyk L, Fahrbach K, Reynolds MW, et al. Adverse events in coronary artery bypass graft (CABG) trials: a systematic review and analysis. Heart 2003;89:767–72.

4. Grüntzig AR, Senning A, Siegenthaler WE. Nonoperative dilatation of coronary-artery stenosis: percutaneous transluminal coronary angioplasty. N Engl J Med 1979;301:61–8.

5. Singh M, Rihal CS, Gersh BJ, et al. Twenty-five-year trends in in-hospital and long-term outcome after percutaneous coronary intervention: a single-institution experience. Circulation 2007; 115:2835–41.

6. Moussa ID, Klein LW, Shah B, et al. Consideration of a new definition of clinically relevant myocardial infarction after coronary revascularization: an expert consensus document from the Society for Cardiovascular Angiography and Interventions (SCAI). J Am Coll Cardiol 2013;62:1563–70.

7. Serruys PW, Silber S, Garg S, et al. Comparison of zotarolimus-eluting and everolimus-eluting coronary stents. N Engl J Med 2010;363:136–46.

8. Lincoff AM, Popma JJ, Ellis SG, et al. Abrupt vessel closure complicating coronary angioplasty: clinical, angiographic and therapeutic profile. J Am Coll Cardiol 1992;19:926–35.

9. Ruygrok PN, Serruys PW. Intracoronary stenting. From concept to custom. Circulation 1996;94: 882–90.

10. Mauri L, Kereiakes DJ, Yeh RW, et al, DAPT Study Investigators. Twelve or 30 months of dual antiplatelet therapy after drug-eluting stents. N Engl J Med 2014;371:2155–66.

11. Sigwart U, Puel J, Mirkovitch V, et al. Intravascular stents to prevent occlusion and restenosis after transluminal angioplasty. N Engl J Med 1987;316: 701–6.

12. Serruys PW, de Jaegere P, Kiemeneij F, et al. A comparison of balloon-expandable-stent implantation with balloon angioplasty in patients with coronary artery disease. Benestent Study Group. N Engl J Med 1994;331:489–95.

13. Fischman DL, Leon MB, Baim DS, et al. A randomized comparison of coronary-stent placement and balloon angioplasty in the treatment of coronary artery disease. Stent Restenosis Study Investigators. N Engl J Med 1994;331: 496–501.

14. Webber BJ, Seguin PG, Burnett DG, et al. Prevalence of and risk factors for autopsy-determined atherosclerosis among US service members, 2001-2011. JAMA 2012;308:2577–83.

15. Chaitman BR, Bourassa MG, Davis K, et al. Angiographic prevalence of high-risk coronary artery disease in patient subsets (CASS). Circulation 1981;64: 360–7.

16. Cho I, Chang HJ, O Hartaigh B, et al. Incremental prognostic utility of coronary CT angiography for asymptomatic patients based upon extent and severity of coronary artery calcium: results from the COronary CT Angiography EvaluatioN For Clinical Outcomes InteRnational Multicenter (CONFIRM) Study. Eur Heart J 2015;36(8):501–8.

17. Muhlestein JB, Lappé DL, Lima JA, et al. Effect of screening for coronary artery disease using CT angiography on mortality and cardiac events in high-risk patients with diabetes: the FACTOR-64 randomized clinical trial. JAMA 2014;312: 2234–43.

18. White CW, Wright CB, Doty DB, et al. Does visual interpretation of the coronary arteriogram predict the physiologic importance of a coronary stenosis? N Engl J Med 1984;310:819–24.

19. CONTRAST (Can cONTrast Injection Better Approximate FFR compAred to Pure reSTing Physiology?). Available at: http://clinicaltrials.gov/ct2/show/NCT02184117. Accessed January 12, 2015.

20. Gould KL, Westcott RJ, Albro PC, et al. Noninvasive assessment of coronary stenoses by myocardial imaging during pharmacologic coronary vasodilation. II. Clinical methodology and feasibility. Am J Cardiol 1978;41:279–87.

21. Wilson RF, White CW. Intracoronary papaverine: an ideal coronary vasodilator for studies of the coronary circulation in conscious humans. Circulation 1986;73:444–51.

22. Wilson RF, Wyche K, Christensen BV, et al. Effects of adenosine on human coronary arterial circulation. Circulation 1990;82:1595–606.

23. Hodgson JM, Williams DO. Superiority of intracoronary papaverine to radiographic contrast for measuring coronary flow reserve in patients with ischemic heart disease. Am Heart J 1987;114: 704–10.

24. Talman CL, Winniford MD, Rossen JD, et al. Polymorphous ventricular tachycardia: a side effect of

intracoronary papaverine. J Am Coll Cardiol 1990; 15:275–8.

25. Pijls NH, Kern MJ, Yock PG, et al. Practice and potential pitfalls of coronary pressure measurement. Catheter Cardiovasc Interv 2000;49:1–16.

26. De Bruyne B, Pijls NH, Barbato E, et al. Intracoronary and intravenous adenosine 5′-triphosphate, adenosine, papaverine, and contrast medium to assess fractional flow reserve in humans. Circulation 2003;107:1877–83.

27. Parham WA, Bouhasin A, Ciaramita JP, et al. Coronary hyperemic dose responses of intracoronary sodium nitroprusside. Circulation 2004;109: 1236–43.

28. Kim W, Jeong MH, Ahn YK, et al. The changes of fractional flow reserve after intracoronary nitrate and Nicorandil injection in coronary artery ectasia. Int J Cardiol 2006;113:250–1.

29. Nair PK, Marroquin OC, Mulukutla SR, et al. Clinical utility of regadenoson for assessing fractional flow reserve. JACC Cardiovasc Interv 2011;4:1085–92.

30. Gregg DE. Coronary circulation in health and disease. Philadelphia: Lea & Febiger; 1950.

31. Marcus ML, Wilson RF, White CW. Methods of measurement of myocardial blood flow in patients: a critical review. Circulation 1987;76:245–53.

32. Khouri EM, Gregg DE. Miniature electromagnetic flow meter applicable to coronary arteries. J Appl Physiol 1963;18:224–7.

33. Benchimol A, Stegall HF, Gartlan JL. New method to measure phasic coronary blood velocity in man. Am Heart J 1971;81:93–101.

34. Cole JS, Hartley CJ. The pulsed Doppler coronary artery catheter preliminary report of a new technique for measuring rapid changes in coronary artery flow velocity in man. Circulation 1977;56:18–25.

35. Marcus M, Wright C, Doty D, et al. Measurements of coronary velocity and reactive hyperemia in the coronary circulation of humans. Circ Res 1981;49: 877–91.

36. Wilson RF, Laughlin DE, Ackell PH, et al. Transluminal, subselective measurement of coronary artery blood flow velocity and vasodilator reserve in man. Circulation 1985;72:82–92.

37. Doucette JW, Corl PD, Payne HM, et al. Validation of a Doppler guide wire for intravascular measurement of coronary artery flow velocity. Circulation 1992;85:1899–911.

38. Segal J, Kern MJ, Scott NA, et al. Alterations of phasic coronary artery flow velocity in humans during percutaneous coronary angioplasty. J Am Coll Cardiol 1992;20:276–86.

39. Kern MJ, Moore JA, Aguirre FV, et al. Determination of angiographic (TIMI grade) blood flow by intracoronary Doppler flow velocity during acute myocardial infarction. Circulation 1996;94: 1545–52.

40. De Bruyne B, Pijls NH, Smith L, et al. Coronary thermodilution to assess flow reserve: experimental validation. Circulation 2001;104:2003–6.

41. Pijls NH, De Bruyne B, Smith L, et al. Coronary thermodilution to assess flow reserve: validation in humans. Circulation 2002;105:2482–6.

42. Aarnoudse W, Van't Veer M, Pijls NH, et al. Direct volumetric blood flow measurement in coronary arteries by thermodilution. J Am Coll Cardiol 2007; 50:2294–304.

43. van der Horst A, Van't Veer M, van der Sligte RA, et al. A combination of thermal methods to assess coronary pressure and flow dynamics with a pressure-sensing guide wire. Med Eng Phys 2013; 35:298–309.

44. Ganz P, Abben R, Friedman PL, et al. Usefulness of transstenotic coronary pressure gradient measurements during diagnostic catheterization. Am J Cardiol 1985;55:910–4.

45. Emanuelsson H, Dohnal M, Lamm C, et al. Initial experiences with a miniaturized pressure transducer during coronary angioplasty. Cathet Cardiovasc Diagn 1991;24:137–43.

46. De Bruyne B, Pijls NH, Paulus WJ, et al. Transstenotic coronary pressure gradient measurement in humans: in vitro and in vivo evaluation of a new pressure monitoring angioplasty guide wire. J Am Coll Cardiol 1993;22:119–26.

47. Pijls NH, De Bruyne B. Coronary pressure. Dordrecht (The Netherlands): Kluwer Academic Publishers; 1997.

48. Banerjee RK, Peelukhana SV, Goswami I. Influence of newly designed monorail pressure sensor catheter on coronary diagnostic parameters: an in vitro study. J Biomech 2014;47:617–24.

49. Thomas DM, Coles GA, Williams JD. What does the renal reserve mean? Kidney Int 1994;45:411–6.

50. Palombo D, Porta C, Peinetti F, et al. Cerebral reserve and indications for shunting in carotid surgery. Cardiovasc Surg 1994;2:32–6.

51. Gatto E, Marchese S, Tedoldi A. Contribution to the interpretation of electrocardiographical tests of coronary reserve: pseudo-improvement of the T wave. Arch Maragliano Patol Clin 1963;19:271–86 [in Italian].

52. Tauchert M. Coronary reserve capacity and maximum oxygen consumption of the human heart. Basic Res Cardiol 1973;68:183–223 [in German].

53. Gould KL, Lipscomb K, Hamilton GW. Physiologic basis for assessing critical coronary stenosis. Instantaneous flow response and regional distribution during coronary hyperemia as measures of coronary flow reserve. Am J Cardiol 1974;33:87–94.

54. Kern MJ. Interventional physiology rounds: case studies in coronary pressure and flow for clinical practice. New York: John Wiley & Sons; 1998.

55. Serruys PW, di Mario C, Piek J, et al. Prognostic value of intracoronary flow velocity and diameter stenosis in assessing the short- and long-term outcomes of coronary balloon angioplasty: the DEBATE Study (Doppler Endpoints Balloon Angioplasty Trial Europe). Circulation 1997;96:3369–77.

56. Serruys PW, de Bruyne B, Carlier S, et al. Randomized comparison of primary stenting and provisional balloon angioplasty guided by flow velocity measurement. Doppler Endpoints Balloon Angioplasty Trial Europe (DEBATE) II Study Group. Circulation 2000;102:2930–7.

57. DEFINE-FLOW (Distal Evaluation of Functional performance with Intravascular sensors to assess the Narrowing Effect – Combined pressure and Doppler FLOW velocity measurements). Available at: https://clinicaltrials.gov/ct2/show/NCT02328820. Accessed January 12, 2015.

58. Kirkeeide RL, Gould KL, Parsel L. Assessment of coronary stenoses by myocardial perfusion imaging during pharmacologic coronary vasodilation. VII. Validation of coronary flow reserve as a single integrated functional measure of stenosis severity reflecting all its geometric dimensions. J Am Coll Cardiol 1986;7:103–13.

59. Johnson NP, Kirkeeide RL, Gould KL. Coronary anatomy to predict physiology: fundamental limits. Circ Cardiovasc Imaging 2013;6:817–32.

60. Gould KL, Johnson NP, Bateman TM, et al. Anatomic versus physiologic assessment of coronary artery disease. Role of coronary flow reserve, fractional flow reserve, and positron emission tomography imaging in revascularization decision-making. J Am Coll Cardiol 2013;62:1639–53.

61. Young DF, Cholvin NR, Kirkeeide RL, et al. Hemodynamics of arterial stenoses at elevated flow rates. Circ Res 1977;41:99–107.

62. Gould KL, Kirkeeide RL, Buchi M. Coronary flow reserve as a physiologic measure of stenosis severity. J Am Coll Cardiol 1990;15:459–74.

63. Pijls NH, van Son JA, Kirkeeide RL, et al. Experimental basis of determining maximum coronary, myocardial, and collateral blood flow by pressure measurements for assessing functional stenosis severity before and after percutaneous transluminal coronary angioplasty. Circulation 1993;87:1354–67.

64. Pijls NH, Bech GJ, el Gamal MI, et al. Quantification of recruitable coronary collateral blood flow in conscious humans and its potential to predict future ischemic events. J Am Coll Cardiol 1995;25:1522–8.

65. De Bruyne B, Pijls NH, Heyndrickx GR, et al. Pressure-derived fractional flow reserve to assess serial epicardial stenoses: theoretical basis and animal validation. Circulation 2000;101:1840–7.

66. De Bruyne B, Hersbach F, Pijls NH, et al. Abnormal epicardial coronary resistance in patients with diffuse atherosclerosis but "normal" coronary angiography. Circulation 2001;104:2401–6.

67. De Bruyne B, Baudhuin T, Melin JA, et al. Coronary flow reserve calculated from pressure measurements in humans. Validation with positron emission tomography. Circulation 1994;89:1013–22.

68. Goff SL, Mazor KM, Ting HH, et al. How cardiologists present the benefits of percutaneous coronary interventions to patients with stable angina: a qualitative analysis. JAMA Intern Med 2014;174:1614–21.

69. Rothberg MB, Scherer L, Kashef MA, et al. The effect of information presentation on beliefs about the benefits of elective percutaneous coronary intervention. JAMA Intern Med 2014;174:1623–9.

70. Gould KL, Johnson NP. Physiologic severity of diffuse coronary artery disease: hidden high risk. Circulation 2015;131:4–6.

71. Gould KL, Johnson NP. Physiologic stenosis severity, binary thinking, revascularization and "hidden reality". Circ Cardiovasc Imaging 2015;8(1).

72. Wong WH, Kirkeeide RL, Gould KL. Computer applications in angiography. In: Collins SM, Skorton DJ, editors. Cardiac imaging and image processing. New York: McGraw Hill; 1986. p. 206–39.

73. Wijns W, Serruys PW, Reiber JH, et al. Quantitative angiography of the left anterior descending coronary artery: correlations with pressure gradient and results of exercise thallium scintigraphy. Circulation 1985;71:273–9.

74. Mancini GB, McGillem MJ, DeBoe SF, et al. The diastolic hyperemic flow versus pressure relation. A new index of coronary stenosis severity and flow reserve. Circulation 1989;80:941–50.

75. Abe M, Tomiyama H, Yoshida H, et al. Diastolic fractional flow reserve to assess the functional severity of moderate coronary artery stenoses: comparison with fractional flow reserve and coronary flow velocity reserve. Circulation 2000;102:2365–70.

76. Meuwissen M, Chamuleau SA, Siebes M, et al. Role of variability in microvascular resistance on fractional flow reserve and coronary blood flow velocity reserve in intermediate coronary lesions. Circulation 2001;103:184–7.

77. Meuwissen M, Siebes M, Chamuleau SA, et al. Hyperemic stenosis resistance index for evaluation of functional coronary lesion severity. Circulation 2002;106:441–6.

78. Ovadia-Blechman Z, Einav S, Zaretsky U, et al. The area of the pressure-flow loop for assessment of arterial stenosis: a new index. Technol Health Care 2002;10:39–56.

79. Brosh D, Higano ST, Slepian MJ, et al. Pulse transmission coefficient: a novel nonhyperemic

parameter for assessing the physiological significance of coronary artery stenoses. J Am Coll Cardiol 2002;39:1012–9.

80. Fearon WF, Balsam LB, Farouque HM, et al. Novel index for invasively assessing the coronary microcirculation. Circulation 2003;107:3129–32.

81. Krams R, Ten Cate FJ, Carlier SG, et al. Diastolic coronary vascular reserve: a new index to detect changes in the coronary microcirculation in hypertrophic cardiomyopathy. J Am Coll Cardiol 2004; 43:670–7.

82. Marques KM, van Eenige MJ, Spruijt HJ, et al. The diastolic flow velocity-pressure gradient relation and dpv50 to assess the hemodynamic significance of coronary stenoses. Am J Physiol Heart Circ Physiol 2006;291:H2630–5.

83. Banerjee RK, Sinha Roy A, Back LH, et al. Characterizing momentum change and viscous loss of a hemodynamic endpoint in assessment of coronary lesions. J Biomech 2007;40:652–62.

84. Sen S, Escaned J, Malik IS, et al. Development and validation of a new adenosine-independent index of stenosis severity from coronary wave-intensity analysis: results of the ADVISE (ADenosine Vasodilator Independent Stenosis Evaluation) study. J Am Coll Cardiol 2012;59:1392–402.

The Concept of Functional Percutaneous Coronary Intervention

Why Physiologic Lesion Assessment Is Integral to Coronary Angiography

Danyaal S. Moin, MD, Allen Jeremias, MD, MSc*

KEYWORDS

• Fractional flow reserve • Coronary artery disease • Coronary revascularization

KEY POINTS

- The majority of revascularization decisions are based solely on the coronary angiogram.
- Anatomic assessments on coronary angiography often times are discordant with hemodynamic stenosis severity.
- Fractional flow reserve (FFR) is a well validated tool to assess coronary stenosis severity.
- The use of FFR to assess coronary stenoses frequently changes revascularization strategies.
- Patients with physiologically insignificant lesions based on FFR do not benefit from revascularization and have an excellent prognosis with optimal medical therapy alone.

INTRODUCTION

The amount of attention directed toward the appropriateness of medical procedures has been increasing steadily in the past years in a rapidly changing health care environment. Increasing amounts of scrutiny have been placed in particular on the use of percutaneous coronary interventions (PCI), because more than 600,000 of these procedures are performed annually within the United States[1] at substantial direct and indirect costs to the health care system. Consequently, a growing amount of oversight has been directed toward the clinical justification of the perceived benefit from many of these revascularization procedures. Given the scope of this problem, there has been a considerable push at both the public and professional levels to assess the "appropriateness" of such procedures, a movement that has even produced action at the congressional level.

Much of this debate was driven by the findings of the landmark Clinical Outcomes Utilizing Revascularization and Aggressive Drug Evaluation (COURAGE) trial.[2] Patients were enrolled into this study based on angiographic stenosis severity by visual assessment, either with a lesion of greater than 70% in the setting of EKG abnormalities or a prior abnormal stress test or a lesion of greater than 80% with concomitant symptoms of classic angina. The overarching conclusion reached in COURAGE was that PCI offered no significant benefit relative to optimal medical therapy (OMT) alone with respect to mortality or myocardial infarction at 5 years in

None of the authors has any conflicts of interest with respect to this review.

Division of Cardiovascular Medicine, Department of Medicine, Stony Brook University Medical Center, Stony Brook, NY, USA

* Corresponding author. Division of Cardiology, Department of Medicine, Health Sciences Center, T16-080, Stony Brook, NY 11794-8160.

E-mail address: allen.jeremias@stonybrookmedicine.edu

the management of patients with stable coronary artery disease (CAD). Importantly, this trial also suggested that the gold standard for the evaluation of ischemia, namely, coronary angiography, was by itself insufficient in identification of lesions that would benefit from PCI. A subsequent metaanalysis of 12 randomized trials including a total of 7182 patients with stable CAD reaffirmed the absence of benefit of PCI against OMT.[3]

APPROPRIATE USE CRITERIA FOR CORONARY REVASCULARIZATION

Appropriate use criteria have been used as a means to identify the appropriateness of both diagnostic tests and therapeutic modalities in a growing number of medical and surgical specialties. Appropriate use criteria with regard to coronary revascularization procedures were formally introduced in February 2009 in a consensus statement released by the American College of Cardiology Appropriate Criteria Task Force, Society for Coronary Angiography and Interventions, Society of Thoracic Surgeons, American Association of Thoracic Surgeons, American Heart Association, and the American Society of Nuclear Cardiology.[4] Applying these criteria in a multicenter prospective analysis of the "appropriateness" of more than 500,000 interventions performed at 1091 centers in the United States from July 2009 to September 2010, Chan and colleagues[5] found that coronary revascularization was nearly always appropriate in the acute setting of ST-elevation myocardial infarctions, non–ST-elevation myocardial infarctions, and high-risk unstable angina (98.6%). In contrast, only 50.4% of interventions performed on patients with stable angina were deemed appropriate when using the novel appropriate use criteria, whereas 11.6% were found inappropriate (with the remainder being in the "uncertain" category). It has to be noted, however, that the study period was shortly after the initial publication of the appropriate use criteria and thus predated the widespread adoption of these criteria. Nevertheless among the inappropriate PCIs, certain characteristics are notable: 72% had low-risk noninvasive tests, 94% lacked high-risk coronary findings on angiography, and only 6% had lesions in the proximal left anterior descending artery. Furthermore, 54% of patients had no symptoms of angina and 96% of this cohort were either on none (42.3%) or only one (52.5%) antianginal medication at the time of PCI. This analysis suggests that the coronary angiogram either alone or in conjunction with noninvasive testing fails to identify lesions suitable for "appropriate" intervention in a substantial number of cases.

The importance of performing PCI on predominately appropriate patients has been demonstrated in a retrospective analysis of 1625 patients that underwent PCI from 2006 to 2007 in the setting of stable angina and suspected CAD.[6] Using the 2009 appropriate use criteria, appropriate revascularization (either coronary artery bypass grafting or PCI) provided a 26.7% decrease in the composite of death and recurrent acute coronary syndrome at 3 years vs. OMT (11.8% vs 16.1%; P = .0087). Additionally, there was a trend toward an increase in adverse events among patients deemed inappropriate for revascularization that nevertheless underwent coronary revascularization (14.2% vs 9.4%; P = .97), albeit not statistically significant owing to the low number of events. Aiming to identify lesions appropriate for revascularization thus has a substantial impact on patient outcomes.

NONINVASIVE ISCHEMIC EVALUATION

Noninvasive testing in the evaluation of patients with stable angina remains the standard of care in the diagnostic workup. Exercise myocardial perfusion imaging and exercise echocardiography have high negative predictive values. The absence of myocardial ischemia on these tests is associated with an excellent prognosis and an annual event rate of 0.45% and 0.54%, respectively, for each modality.[7] Similarly, a metaanalysis of 19 studies demonstrated that a normal or low-risk single photon emission CT result was associated with a 0.6% annual risk of major cardiac events.[8] These data demonstrate that, at a population level, noninvasive testing provides a robust means of risk stratification of patients with suspected CAD. However, in individual cases, noninvasive testing may prove to be less reliable, perhaps providing an explanation for the poor use of noninvasive testing before cardiac catheterization. A retrospective analysis of 23,887 patients insured by Medicare aged 65 or older found that only 44.5% underwent stress testing in the 90 days preceding elective PCI.[9] Subgroup analyses demonstrate that the highest volume providers (>150 PCIs annually) were least likely to perform stress testing before PCI (odds ratio, 0.84; 95% CI, 0.77–0.93). In addition, use of stress testing in academic teaching hospitals was similar to that in the overall population, suggesting that the use of noninvasive testing is independent of academic or teaching status. In a more contemporary analysis, Dehmer and colleagues[10] demonstrated a similarly low rate of noninvasive testing before PCI among almost 1 million patients in the National Cardiovascular Disease Registry database. Given the limitations of noninvasive testing in individual patients and the lack of its universal use before cardiac catheterization, it is not surprising that clinical decisions with respect to revascularization are based most frequently on anatomic variables (the coronary angiogram) alone. Anatomic lesion severity, however, may not always correlate well with coronary hemodynamics and the presence of myocardial ischemia.

ANATOMIC LESION SEVERITY AND CORONARY HEMODYNAMICS

Based on animal models of myocardial ischemia, Gould[11] elegantly described the relationship between coronary stenosis severity and myocardial blood flow. In this classic experiment, the translesional decrease in pressure is a function of stenosis severity and coronary flow velocity. As the severity of the stenosis increases, a compensatory dilatation of the microcirculation occurs in an effort to maintain consistent myocardial perfusion with a decrease in perfusion pressure only in the most severe lesions.[12] As a result of this complex interplay between the severity of epicardial stenosis and myocardial blood flow, the purely anatomic assessment of any given coronary stenosis may be insufficient to determine its impact on myocardial perfusion and potential ischemia.

Evidence from multiple recent trials is emerging that describe the discrepancy between angiographic coronary stenosis severity and its functional impact on myocardial ischemia. Among the 509 patients in the Fractional Flow Reserve versus Angiography for Multivessel Evaluation (FAME) study with angiographically detected multivessel CAD (a total of 1329 stenoses), only 46% had functional multivessel disease.[13] This means that fewer than one-half of coronary stenoses deemed "significant" on angiography proved to be of hemodynamic consequence causing ischemia at the level of the myocardium. The vast majority of intermediate lesions (defined as 50%–70% stenosis severity) were associated with "negative" fractional flow reserve (FFR) results (65%). Even more striking, angiographically critical lesions (stenosis severity of 71%–90%) still had a 20% rate of negative FFR measurements. Based on this evidence, a recent expert consensus statement on the use of FFR recommended expanding its use beyond the intermediate lesion to the full spectrum of coronary stenoses up to 90% in severity.[14]

A recent study demonstrated the discrepancy between angiographic lesion assessment and physiologic stenosis severity. Using data from the Registrie Francais de la Fractional Flow Reserve, the role of FFR in clinical decision making was investigated in 1075 patients from 20 French centers.[15] Treating physicians were asked to make a decision regarding coronary revascularization or medical management after performing the diagnostic angiogram according to their usual clinical practice. FFR measurements were then performed of all lesions. Overall, the number of patients categorized into medical management, PCI, and bypass surgery groups was not substantially different a priori and after FFR evaluation (55% vs 58%, 38% vs 32%, and 7% vs 10%, respectively). However, when evaluated at an individual patient level, FFR altered the revascularization strategy in 43% of cases with roughly equal proportions in each subset (Fig. 1). Interestingly, noninvasive

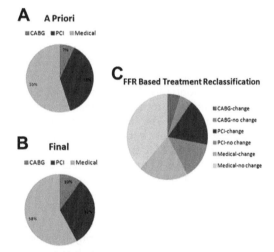

Fig. 1. Relative proportions of revascularization decisions made before (A) and after (B) performing fractional flow reserve (FFR) measurements. There was only a small overall statistical difference in the grouping when FFR was incorporated ($P = .02$) into revascularization decisions. At the individual patient level, however, there were substantial changes (C) in treatment strategy from the a priori to FFR based revascularization strategies with almost half the patients requiring reclassification. CABG, coronary artery bypass grafting; PCI, percutaneous coronary intervention. (Data from Van Belle E, Rioufol G, Pouillot C, et al. Outcome impact of coronary revascularization strategy reclassification with fractional flow reserve at time of diagnostic angiography: insights from a large French multicenter fractional flow reserve registry. Circulation 2014;129(2):173–85.)

testing before coronary angiography was only modestly predictive when compared with FFR in determining treatment classification in the subgroup of patients that had prior testing. Furthermore, the incidence of major cardiac events was no different in reclassified patients versus those with concordant angiographic and FFR findings (11.2% vs 11.9%; $P = .78$).

Factors that led to discordance between conventional angiography and FFR were assessed in a 1000-patient, prospective cohort analysis by Park and colleagues.[16] "Mismatches" were defined in this study as lesions with greater than 50% diameter stenoses but negative FFR measurements (ie, >0.80). Conversely, "reverse mismatches" involved lesions with less than 50% diameter stenoses with an FFR of 0.80 or less. Mismatches occurred more frequently in lesions outside the left main coronary artery (57% vs 35%; $P = .032$), whereas reverse mismatches were more common within the left main coronary artery (40% vs 16%; $P<.001$).

INVASIVE EVALUATION OF ISCHEMIA

In 2012, the appropriate use criteria were expanded to incorporate recommendations regarding diagnostic cardiac catheterizations.[17] Notable within the document was the recommendation of the use of FFR as an "adjunct to coronary angiography for the determination of lesion severity and to assist in decisions about revascularization." The incorporation of FFR into these recommendations was largely driven by findings of the FAME study.[18] This clinical trial of 1015 patients with multivessel CAD demonstrated than an FFR based revascularization strategy significantly reduced the 1 year rate of major adverse cardiac events (13.2% vs 18.3%; $P = .02$) compared with a strategy based on visual lesion assessment by coronary angiography. This treatment difference persisted over longer term follow-up,[19] with a significant reduction of death and myocardial infarction in the FFR-guided group (8.4% vs 12.9%; $P = .02$) at 2 years.

The improved clinical outcomes observed in the FAME study are based largely on accurately identifying lesions that may benefit from revascularization and avoiding the risk of coronary revascularization in stenoses that are unlikely to benefit. However, this strategy can only be successful if "FFR-negative" lesions have a low enough event rate over time when treated with medical therapy alone. Berger and colleagues[20] prospectively analyzed 102 patients with multivessel CAD in whom multivessel PCI was being considered. Among these patients, at least 1 vessel underwent PCI and the other(s) were deferred when FFR was greater than 0.75. With a mean follow-up of 29 months, major adverse cardiac events occurred in 22 discrete vessels. Of those vessels, only 8 were coronary arteries that did not have prior PCI and the remaining 14 culprit arteries were associated with previously revascularized vessels. These findings were further expounded when FFR was performed in a prospective study of 852 patients with intermediate lesions (30%–70%) of the proximal left anterior descending artery on coronary angiography.[21] Hemodynamically significant (FFR <0.80) lesions were revascularized, whereas the remainder were treated with OMT. The 5-year mortality was similar between this medically treated group and a separate control group without CAD that was matched or age and gender (92.9% vs 89.6%; $P = .74$). Additionally, patients enrolled in FAME with lesions that were deferred based on FFR at the time of cardiac catheterization had only a 0.2% rate of myocardial infarction and a 3.2% rate of revascularization over 2 years of follow-up.[19]

The DEFER study[22] validated the role of FFR in patients scheduled for elective PCI of intermediate grade (>50%) stenoses in 325 patients without any evidence of inducible ischemia on noninvasive testing. Patients were randomized into 2 groups before acquisition of FFR data, one in which PCI would be deferred pending FFR results and another in which PCI would be performed irrespective of FFR findings. As expected, patients with myocardial ischemia based on the FFR measurement (<0.75) had a higher incidence of cardiovascular events at 1 year compared with patients without ischemia by FFR. In patients who were randomized to PCI versus medical management without evidence of ischemia (FFR >0.75), there was no difference in event-free survival at 2 years[22] or 5 years[23] (80% vs 73%; $P = .52$) with a trend toward higher event-free survival among the medically treated patients.

FRACTIONAL FLOW RESERVE AS AN INTEGRAL PART OF CORONARY ANGIOGRAPHY

The ability of FFR to further refine the angiographic assessment of lesion severity has been demonstrated in numerous studies. One such example is the use of the 'Synergy Between Percutaneous Coronary Intervention with Taxus and Cardiac Surgery' (SYNTAX) score, a prognostic tool used in patients with multivessel

CAD to aid in revascularization strategies that is predicated solely on anatomic characteristics obtained during routine angiography. Nam and colleagues[24] postulated that a 'functional' SYN-TAX score, defined as one that only incorporates coronary lesions that are capable of producing ischemia (FFR <0.80), may be of greater prognostic and clinical value than the traditional SYN-TAX score. Among a 497-patient subset of the FAME study, the adjusted SYNTAX score not only better predicted the incidence of major adverse cardiac events, but also facilitated reclassification of patients to a lower risk category in 32% of the patient population. The clinical impact of this reclassification is observed by the fact that patients that were reclassified from a high-risk group under the conventional SYNTAX scoring to a medium- or low-risk group with the "functional" SYNTAX score had a significantly lower rate of death, myocardial infarction, or repeat revascularization at 1 year compared with those who remained within the high-risk category (11.3% vs 26.7%; P = .028).

Although most studies evaluate the impact of FFR in a dichotomous fashion (ie, FFR "positive" or "negative" by using a single cut-off point, most commonly 0.80 or 0.75), it makes intuitive sense that FFR represents a range of biological variables and that lower FFR values represent a larger amount of ischemia or greater area at risk. Under that assumption, coronary stenoses that produce high FFR values should demonstrate no or minimal myocardial ischemia and outcomes should be excellent with OMT alone. On the other hand, lesions with very low FFR values should be associated with a large amount of myocardial ischemia, either because the lesion is severely stenotic or because the coronary artery under evaluation is supplying a large amount of myocardium. In theory, the benefit of coronary revascularization should be roughly proportional the FFR value such that revascularization derives greater benefit in patients with lower FFR values. Johnson and colleagues[25] examined this question in a metaanalysis combining data from all FFR outcome trials at both the study level (eg, cohort data) and patient level. Regression analyses were performed at both levels to identify an FFR threshold at which superiority is established for either medical therapy or revascularization in reducing death, myocardial infarction, or target vessel and lesion revascularization at 1 year. In the cohort model, medical therapy was superior to revascularization in a continuous manner at FFR values above 0.75 with the relationship reversing at FFR values below that

threshold. As hypothesized, a greater treatment benefit was indeed observed at lower FFR levels.

A NEW APPROACH OF FUNCTIONAL ANGIOGRAPHY

Despite the evidence that FFR as an adjunct to coronary angiography has the ability to identify ischemia-producing stenoses that warrant revascularization and also identify lesions that do not produce sufficient myocardial ischemia to justify the risk of a revascularization procedure, physiologic lesion assessment in the cardiac catheterization laboratory is severely underused. Analysis of 61,874 attempted coronary interventions of intermediate stenoses in the CathPCI registry found that FFR was only used in 6.1% of cases.[26] In that same registry, FFR was used more often in academic medical centers and in patients with either an equivocal or negative stress test. Ultimately, the question to be asked is how to perform coronary angiography so as to provide the best likelihood of performing PCI on ischemia-producing lesions and avoiding PCI on lesions that can be treated effectively with OMT.

Park and colleagues[27] have posited the notion of the "functional angioplasty," a strategy that incorporates FFR into revascularization decisions. The basic concept of that strategy is that revascularization should be justified by instability of the stenosis in question (eg, acute coronary syndrome) or by objective evidence of myocardial ischemia as a result of a specific lesion rather than a decision based on the anatomic assessment provided by the coronary angiogram. In this strategy, patients with stable angina and myocardial ischemia on prior noninvasive testing should undergo PCI if a coronary stenosis is discovered in a "concordant" territory (eg, anterior ischemia on a stress test in the presence of a lesion in the left anterior descending artery). However, if the anatomic stenosis is in a discordant territory or noninvasive testing was not performed before angiography, hemodynamic evaluation of the stenosis is recommended to assist with further decision making. PCI should then only be performed if the stenosis is found to be of hemodynamic significance by FFR. Similarly, in patients undergoing coronary angiography in the setting of an acute coronary syndrome, the significance of a nonculprit stenosis can potentially be investigated with the use of FFR if revascularization is being considered of that nonculprit lesion. A summary of indications for hemodynamic stenosis evaluation by coronary physiology is provided in Table 1.

Table 1
Recommendations regarding the use of FFR from a consensus statement of the Society of Coronary Angiography and Interventions

Clinical Setting	Recommendation
Stable ischemic heart disease	Evaluation of intermediate (50%–70%) and severe (<90%) coronary stenoses when noninvasive testing is contraindicated, discordant, nondiagnostic, or unavailable
	PCI of lesions with FFR of <0.80 improves symptoms and decreases repeat revascularization relative to medical therapy
	Medical therapy is indicated for angiographically intermediate stenoses when FFR >0.80
Multivessel CAD	FFR guided PCI improves clinical outcomes relative to an angiography-based strategy
	"Functional" SYNTAX scoring to reclassify patients, potentially changing decision of CABG vs PCI

Abbreviations: CABG, coronary artery bypass grafting; FFR, fractional flow reserve; PCI, percutaneous coronary intervention.
　　Lotfi A, Jeremias A, Fearon WF, et al. Expert consensus statement on the use of fractional flow reserve, intravascular ultrasound, and optical coherence tomography. Catheter Cardiovasc Interv 2014;83(4):509–18.

SUMMARY

The clinical indication for coronary revascularization should not be based on anatomic factors provided by the coronary angiogram in a vacuum. The appropriate use criteria use a combination of anatomy, symptoms, and functional testing as its basic pillars of decision making. Similarly, numerous studies using coronary physiology for clinical decision making have demonstrated superior outcomes when compared with an anatomy-based strategy. The use of angiography alone to make decisions about revascularization carries the dual risk of performing inappropriate PCIs and also deferring PCI on lesions that would have otherwise benefited from revascularization. Unfortunately, the vast majority of PCI procedures performed in the current era continue to be driven by anatomic assessments of lesion severity. The clinical adoption of a "functional" PCI strategy that uses FFR as an integral component of the diagnostic coronary angiogram as a means to provide an objective ischemia assessment is essential to better guide revascularization decisions in the future.

REFERENCES

1. Kozak LJ, Lees KA, DeFrances CJ. National Hospital Discharge Survey: 2003 annual summary with detailed diagnosis and procedure data. Vital Health Stat 13 2006;(160):1–206.
2. Boden WE, O'Rourke RA, Teo KK, et al. Optimal medical therapy with or without PCI for stable coronary disease. N Engl J Med 2007;356(15):1503–16.
3. Pursnani S, Korley F, Gopaul R, et al. Percutaneous coronary intervention versus optimal medical therapy in stable coronary artery disease: a systematic review and meta-analysis of randomized clinical trials. Circ Cardiovasc Interv 2012;5(4):476–90.
4. Patel MR, Dehmer GJ, Hirshfeld JW, et al. ACCF/SCAI/STS/AATS/AHA/ASNC 2009 appropriateness criteria for coronary revascularization: a report by the American College of Cardiology Foundation Appropriateness Criteria Task Force, Society for Cardiovascular Angiography and Interventions, Society of Thoracic Surgeons, American Association for Thoracic Surgery, American Heart Association, and the American Society of Nuclear Cardiology Endorsed by the American Society of Echocardiography, the Heart Failure Society of America, and the Society of Cardiovascular Computed Tomography. J Am Coll Cardiol 2009; 53(6):530–53.
5. Chan PS, Patel MR, Klein LW, et al. Appropriateness of percutaneous coronary intervention. JAMA 2011;306(1):53–61.
6. Ko DT, Guo H, Wijeysundera HC, et al. Assessing the association of appropriateness of coronary revascularization and clinical outcomes for patients with stable coronary artery disease. J Am Coll Cardiol 2012;60(19):1876–84.
7. Metz LD, Beattie M, Hom R, et al. The prognostic value of normal exercise myocardial perfusion imaging and exercise echocardiography: a meta-analysis. J Am Coll Cardiol 2007;49(2):227–37.
8. Shaw LJ, Iskandrian AE. Prognostic value of gated myocardial perfusion SPECT. J Nucl Cardiol 2004; 11(2):171–85.
9. Lin GA, Dudley RA, Lucas FL, et al. Frequency of stress testing to document ischemia prior to

elective percutaneous coronary intervention. JAMA 2008;300(15):1765–73.

10. Dehmer GJ, Weaver D, Roe MT, et al. A contemporary view of diagnostic cardiac catheterization and percutaneous coronary intervention in the United States: a report from the CathPCI Registry of the National Cardiovascular Data Registry, 2010 through June 2011. J Am Coll Cardiol 2012;60(20): 2017–31.

11. Gould KL. Pressure-flow characteristics of coronary stenoses in unsedated dogs at rest and during coronary vasodilation. Circ Res 1978;43(2):242–53.

12. Uren NG, Melin JA, De Bruyne B, et al. Relation between myocardial blood flow and the severity of coronary-artery stenosis. N Engl J Med 1994; 330(25):1782–8.

13. Tonino PA, Fearon WF, De Bruyne B, et al. Angiographic versus functional severity of coronary artery stenoses in the FAME study fractional flow reserve versus angiography in multivessel evaluation. J Am Coll Cardiol 2010;55(25):2816–21.

14. Lotfi A, Jeremias A, Fearon WF, et al. Expert consensus statement on the use of fractional flow reserve, intravascular ultrasound, and optical coherence tomography. Catheter Cardiovasc Interv 2014;83(4):509–18.

15. Van Belle E, Rioufol G, Pouillot C, et al. Outcome impact of coronary revascularization strategy reclassification with fractional flow reserve at time of diagnostic angiography: insights from a large French multicenter fractional flow reserve registry. Circulation 2014;129(2):173–85.

16. Park SJ, Kang SJ, Ahn JM, et al. Visual-functional mismatch between coronary angiography and fractional flow reserve. JACC Cardiovasc Interv 2012; 5(10):1029–36.

17. Patel MR, Bailey SR, Bonow RO, et al. ACCF/SCAI/ AATS/AHA/ASE/ASNC/HFSA/HRS/SCCM/SCCT/ SCMR/STS 2012 appropriate use criteria for diagnostic catheterization: a report of the American College of Cardiology Foundation Appropriate Use Criteria Task Force, Society for Cardiovascular Angiography and Interventions, American Association for Thoracic Surgery, American Heart Association, American Society of Echocardiography, American Society of Nuclear Cardiology, Heart Failure Society of America, Heart Rhythm Society, Society of Critical Care Medicine, Society of Cardiovascular Computed Tomography, Society for Cardiovascular Magnetic Resonance, and Society

of Thoracic Surgeons. J Am Coll Cardiol 2012; 59(22):1995–2027.

18. Tonino PA, De Bruyne B, Pijls NH, et al. Fractional flow reserve versus angiography for guiding percutaneous coronary intervention. N Engl J Med 2009; 360(3):213–24.

19. Pijls NH, Fearon WF, Tonino PA, et al. Fractional flow reserve versus angiography for guiding percutaneous coronary intervention in patients with multivessel coronary artery disease: 2-year follow-up of the FAME (Fractional Flow Reserve Versus Angiography for Multivessel Evaluation) study. J Am Coll Cardiol 2010;56(3):177–84.

20. Berger A, Botman KJ, MacCarthy PA, et al. Long-term clinical outcome after fractional flow reserve-guided percutaneous coronary intervention in patients with multivessel disease. J Am Coll Cardiol 2005;46(3):438–42.

21. Muller O, Mangiacapra F, Ntalianis A, et al. Long-term follow-up after fractional flow reserve-guided treatment strategy in patients with an isolated proximal left anterior descending coronary artery stenosis. JACC Cardiovasc Interv 2011;4(11):1175–82.

22. Bech GJ, De Bruyne B, Pijls NH, et al. Fractional flow reserve to determine the appropriateness of angioplasty in moderate coronary stenosis: a randomized trial. Circulation 2001;103(24):2928–34.

23. Pijls NH, van Schaardenburgh P, Manoharan G, et al. Percutaneous coronary intervention of functionally nonsignificant stenosis: 5-year follow-up of the DEFER Study. J Am Coll Cardiol 2007;49(21):2105–11.

24. Nam CW, Mangiacapra F, Entjes R, et al. Functional SYNTAX score for risk assessment in multivessel coronary artery disease. J Am Coll Cardiol 2011; 58(12):1211–8.

25. Johnson NP, Tóth GG, Lai D, et al. Prognostic value of fractional flow reserve: linking physiologic severity to clinical outcomes. J Am Coll Cardiol 2014;64(16):1641–54.

26. Dattilo PB, Prasad A, Honeycutt E, et al. Contemporary patterns of fractional flow reserve and intravascular ultrasound use among patients undergoing percutaneous coronary intervention in the United States: insights from the National Cardiovascular Data Registry. J Am Coll Cardiol 2012;60(22):2337–9.

27. Park SJ, Ahn JM, Kang SJ. Paradigm shift to functional angioplasty: new insights for fractional flow reserve- and intravascular ultrasound-guided percutaneous coronary intervention. Circulation 2011; 124(8):951–7.

Limitations and Pitfalls of Fractional Flow Reserve Measurements and Adenosine-Induced Hyperemia

Arnold H. Seto, MD, MPA*, David Tehrani, MD, MS, Morton J. Kern, MD

KEYWORDS

- Fractional flow reserve • Limitations • Ischemic coronary artery disease • Coronary stenosis
- Adenosine-induced hyperemia

KEY POINTS

- Fractional flow reserve (FFR) provides a reliable lesion-specific and vessel-specific assessment of the functional significance (ischemic potential) of coronary stenoses.
- Operators must be aware of multiple technical pitfalls of measurement including wire drift, guide catheter damping, beat-to-beat variation, and wire artifacts.
- Adenosine is associated with dynamic and variable hemodynamic responses that can complicate the interpretation of FFR.
- FFR is measured clinically without regard to central venous pressure, which may become relevant in certain patient subgroups.
- Specific clinical settings that may complicate FFR measurement include multivessel disease, acute myocardial infarction, and left main stenosis.

INTRODUCTION

Coronary physiologic assessment addresses the well-known limitations of coronary angiography in determining the clinical significance of intermediate lesions. FFR is increasingly accepted as the gold standard for determining the ischemic potential of coronary lesions and guiding percutaneous coronary intervention (PCI). FFR is an index of the functional significance of coronary stenosis defined as the maximal flow in a vessel in the presence of a stenosis divided by the maximal flow in the theoretic absence of the stenosis. Assuming flow is linearly related to pressure during hyperemia, the translesional pressure ratio serves as a surrogate for the percent of normal flow. The derivation of FFR, Pd − Pv/Pa − Pv, during maximal hyperemia, describes the ischemic potential of the lesion (Pd is the pressure distal to a stenosis, measured by a pressure guide wire, and Pa is the pressure proximal, measured by the pressure transducer on the guiding catheter; the effect of central venous pressure, Pv, is assumed to be clinically negligible).[1]

BASIC PRINCIPLES AND PREREQUISITES

FFR is a technique that is simple to learn yet can be difficult to master because of several caveats that can give inaccurate pressure measurements.

Conflicts of interest: Dr A. Seto is a speaker for Volcano. Dr M. Kern is a speaker for Volcano and St. Jude Medical, and a consultant to Acist Medical and Opsens Medical. No other conflicts.
Department of Medicine, Long Beach Veterans Affairs Medical Center, 5901 East 7th Street 111C, Long Beach, CA 90822, USA
* Corresponding author.
E-mail address: arnoldseto@yahoo.com

Following are the steps that are essential to collect accurate FFR measurements and minimize the risk of error:

1. Administer anticoagulant (usually intravenous [IV] heparin) and intracoronary (IC) nitroglycerin (100- to 200-µg bolus) before insertion of the guide wire.
2. Calibrate the pressure guide wire to the system's analyzer: zero to atmospheric pressure outside of the body. Tighten all pressure tubing connections.
3. Insert the pressure guide wire into the guide catheter and match the wire/guide catheter pressures in the aorta. This process requires removing the needle introducer, tightening the Y-connector (Tuohy-Borst), and flushing the catheter with saline.
4. Advance the wire across the lesion 2 to 3 cm distal to the coronary lesion. Again, this requires removing the needle introducer, tightening the Y-connector, and flushing the catheter with saline.
5. Induce maximal hyperemia with IV adenosine (140 µg/kg/min) or IC bolus of adenosine (20–30 µg for the right coronary artery [RCA] or 60–100 µg for the left coronary artery).
6. When using IC adenosine, measure FFR as the lowest Pd/Pa after hyperemia is induced

(usually 15–20 seconds after injection). When using IV adenosine, measure FFR after 1.5 to 3 minutes of infusion and do not accept pressure for calculations until stable hyperemia is seen for at least several seconds.
7. Confirm the absence of signal drift with pressure wire pullback into the guide. Equal pressure readings indicate wire signal stability.

PITFALLS OF FRACTIONAL FLOW RESERVE MEASUREMENTS
Mechanical Issues: Transducers, Zeros, Connections

Measurement of aortic pressure through a fluid-filled guide catheter is subject to technical issues such as loose connections, leak in guide connections, and improper zeroing. Improper leveling of the systemic pressure transducer can overestimate or underestimate aortic pressure. Loose connections and malfunctioning pressure transducers can generate abnormal or moving systemic pressure measurements, mimicking wire drift. Most commonly, the Y-connector or Tuohy-Borst connector may be inadequately tightened, or the needle introducer left in during measurement or normalization of pressures, leading to a decrease in measured aortic pressure (**Fig. 1**). Finally, a saline flush before any pressure measurement clears

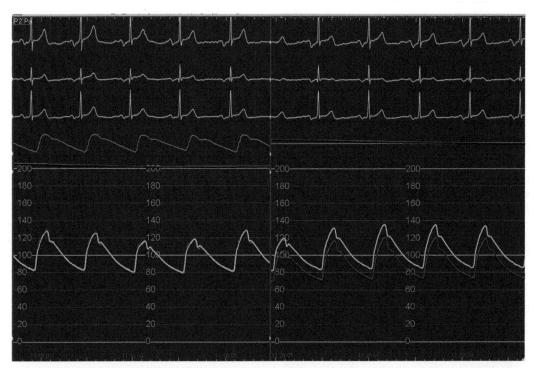

Fig. 1. Loose connections. Equalized Pa and Pd pressures (*left panel*) becomes unequal when the Tuohy-Borst introducer is not tightened (*right panel*), causing partial loss of aortic pressure. Leaving a needle introducer in place causes a similar loss of pressure.

blood and radiographic contrast from the guide catheter, reducing the risk of a damped aortic pressure waveform (Fig. 2).

Beat-to-Beat Variation

Physiologic pressure measurements frequently vary from one beat to another. These variations can result from spontaneous respiration, coughing (Fig. 3), arrhythmias (Fig. 4), or exaggerated respiratory activity (eg, sleep apnea). The default setting for the commercial FFR software from Volcano Corp and St. Jude Medical is to take the lowest value of Pd/Pa over a single beat, resulting in an underestimated FFR. The authors and other investigators recommend changing the settings of the software to measure the 3-beat average FFR to minimize the impact of beat-to-beat variation (Fig. 5).

Damping of Pressure by Guiding Catheter

FFR measurement relies on transduction of aortic pressure through the guide catheter. Owing to the guide catheter size relative to the aortic coronary ostium, it is possible for the guide to create a partial obstruction and an additional gradient between the aorta and the proximal coronary artery, resulting in a distorted aortic waveform known as damping. Damping is most common with larger guiding catheters (8F), but it can also occur with 6F guide catheters in the setting of small coronary ostia or when the catheter is not coaxial with the artery. Extra backup guides are most commonly associated with damping, but any catheter that is deeply seated can create aortic pressure damping. The use of guide extenders (Guideliner [Vascular

Solutions, Minneapolis, MN], Guidezilla [Boston Scientific, Marlborough, MA]) would also be expected to create this effect.

When damping occurs, the guide catheter no longer reflects the aortic pressure; rather it reflects a proximal coronary pressure with an additional gradient from the guide. Aortic pressure damping lowers the measured Pa, underestimating the hyperemic gradient and lesion severity while overestimating the true FFR value (Fig. 6). The guiding catheter may also blunt maximum blood flow through the artery, causing an ischemic process in itself. This phenomenon is best recognized by careful visual examination of the aortic pressure waveform and best prevented by disengaging the guide catheter from the ostium at the time of measurement.

Catheters with Side Holes

Use of guide catheters with side holes in cases of aortic pressure damping introduces a potential source of error in that a pressure gradient through the guide side holes may be formed. A catheter with side holes may produce a pressure reading that is a combination of the aortic and coronary pressures, leading to a higher recorded value than the true proximal coronary pressure (Fig. 7).[2] The additional gradient may not be detected until hyperemia has occurred, and hence FFR may be underestimated. If a guiding catheter with side holes is to be used, then it is mandatory to disengage the catheter from the coronary ostium before pressure measurements are made. The use of IC adenosine is not advised, given that part of the drug may be delivered into the aorta.

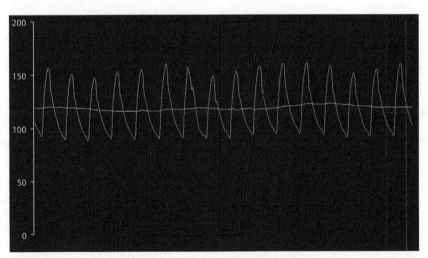

Fig. 2. Contrast damping. Equalized Pa and Pd pressures (*left*) become unequal after an injection of radiographic contrast causes damping of the Pa waveform (*right*) owing to the viscosity of the contrast medium; this can also occur with blood, and is accentuated by the use of small-caliber guides or diagnostic catheters.

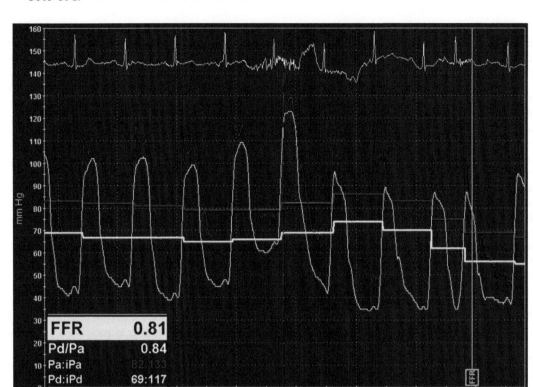

Fig. 3. Cough. Transient rise in both Pd and Pa in response to coughing reflex (evident on electrocardiographic tracing) increasing intrathoracic pressure. Pd, distal pressure; Pa, aortic pressure.

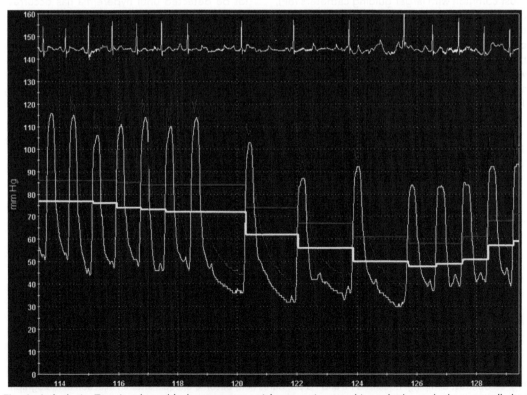

Fig. 4. Arrhythmia. Transient heart block, premature atrial contractions, and irregular heart rhythms may all alter the Pd/Pa relationship.

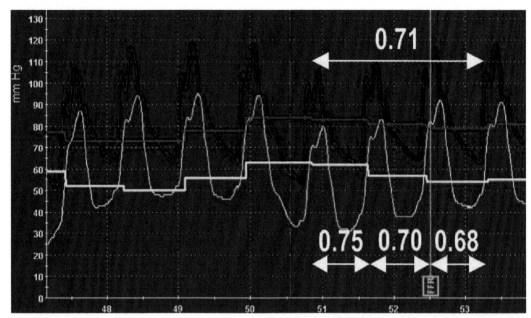

Fig. 5. Measurement of FFR by 1-beat versus 3-beat averages. The single-beat FFR varies from 0.68 to 0.75, whereas the 3-beat average FFR attenuates these fluctuations and is preferred. (*From* Seto AH, Tehrani DM, Bharmal MI, et al. Variations of coronary hemodynamic responses to intravenous adenosine infusion: implications for fractional flow reserve measurements. Catheter Cardiovasc Interv 2014;84(3):422; with permission.)

Guide Wire Whipping Phenomenon

An uncommon artifact of the guide wire sensor is the phenomenon of whipping. During cardiac contraction, the guide wire sensor may hit a moving coronary wall and produce an exaggerated and sharp increase in the pressure signal (Fig. 8). While this artifact increases the recorded coronary pressure, the nonphysiologic waveform is easily recognized. Correction of the whipping artifact is performed by withdrawing or advancing the wire a few millimeters and avoiding placement of the wire into small side branches.

Wire Signal Drift

All piezoelectric pressure sensors are subject to electronic signal offset or drift during a procedure. Signal stability is confirmed by checking the matching of aortic and guide wire pressures at the guide catheter before and after the measurements. On occasion, after inserting the guide wire across a lesion, a resting gradient with the aortic pressure may be noted. Several clues suggest that it is not a true pressure gradient and is instead the result of signal drift, including (1) distal pressure is higher than aortic pressure, (2) the distal pressure signal is unstable and continues to drift higher or lower (Fig. 9), or (3) distal pressure is lower than aortic pressure but retains the identical waveform characteristics. A true significant stenosis acts like a high-frequency filter and obscures transmission of high-frequency signals responsible for the

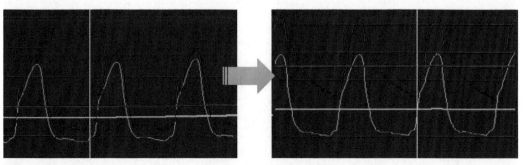

Fig. 6. Guide catheter damping. When oversized or deep seated, a guide catheter can create a damped Pa waveform (*left panel*) that lacks a dicrotic notch. Disengagement of the guide reveals the true higher aortic pressure waveform (*right panel*).

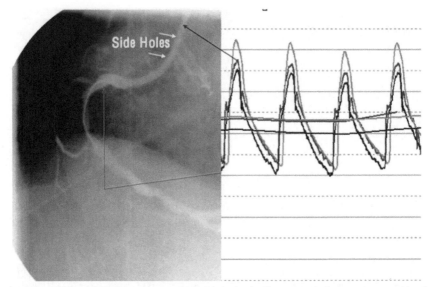

Fig. 7. Confounding effects of guiding catheters with side holes (*yellow arrows*). Pa is represented by the red pressure wave, whereas Pd is represented by the blue pressure wave. The femoral artery pressure (*green*) is also recorded by the side arm of the arterial sheath. The sensor has been advanced to the tip of the guiding catheter, and hyperemia has been induced. A gradient has developed between the femoral pressure and the Pa.

dicrotic notch in the aortic pressure. Therefore, when a translesional pressure gradient is present, but pressure recordings are identical in shape, signal drift should be suspected.

Signal drift occurs most commonly with the following:

1. Disconnection/reconnection of the wire, especially after PCI.
2. Prolonged use of the wire and exposure to blood.

3. Older generations (before 2013) of pressure wires. Note that fiber-optic wires and catheters have less signal drift than piezoelectric sensors.

Wire Spasm and Pseudostenosis

Like any coronary guide wire, passing of a coronary pressure guide wire can induce vasoconstriction and spasm. Coronary spasm narrows the artery and thus can generate a pressure gradient consistent with a physiologic stenosis.

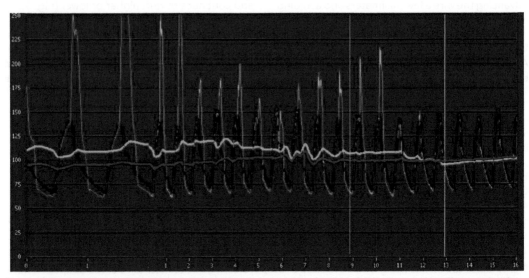

Fig. 8. Wire sensor whip. When the guide wire sensor is in direct contact with the coronary wall or myocardium, brief spikes in the pressure signal are measured by the wire.

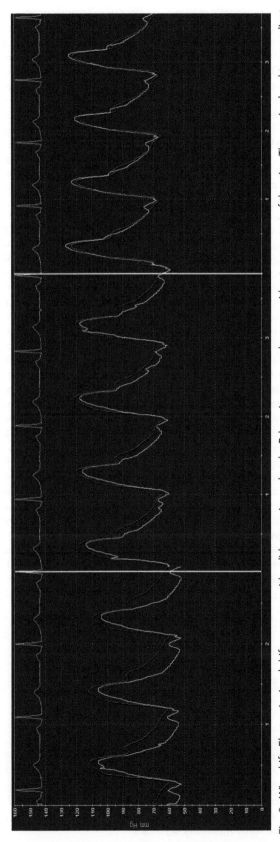

Fig. 9. Wire drift. Electronic signal drift can occur with solid-state wires, whereby Pd can increase or decrease without movement of the wire. The maximal and true gradient (*left panel*) decreases (*center panel*) and even reverses with wire drift (*right panel*), without any movement of the wire or change in the waveform.

To demonstrate that such a vasospastic stenosis is reversible, IC nitroglycerin (100–400 μg) should be given before measuring FFR. Even in the relatively hypotensive patient (systolic pressure 90–100 mm Hg), 50–100 μg of IC nitroglycerin is generally safe and well tolerated.

Guide wires of all types can also create straightening artifacts in tortuous vessels, producing the so-called accordion effect (Fig. 10). This phenomenon occurs especially in the RCA and with the use of stiffer wires or catheters. Guide wire straightening can create temporary obstructions or kinking that can decrease the FFR. Pseudostenoses are detected and tested by observing the lesion after pulling back on the guide wire to the guide, or having only the most flexible wire tip portion in the tortuous section. In the presence of significant tortuosity and straightening with potential pseudostenosis, an accurate FFR may be unmeasurable with available pressure wires.

Effect of Hydrostatic Pressure

One assumption of comparing Pd with Pa is that both the distal and proximal pressures are at the same level in the heart relative to the pressure transducer; this is certainly the case at the time of equalization at the guide catheter tip. However, when the wire is advanced into the coronary circulation, there may be a small change in its position relative to the heart, which can result in a small change in pressure measured due to hydrostatic forces (eg, gravity). This phenomenon occurs primarily in the distal RCA, posterior descending artery, and distal circumflex artery and may result in a small 0.01 to 0.04 increase in FFR measurement. This effect is particularly evident in normal vessels in which the resting Pd/Pa may be as high as 1.04. Pullback into the guide confirms the absence of wire signal drift and the physiologic basis of the change in distal pressure.

Pressure Recovery

In the setting of a severe stenosis in a comparably small distal vessel, the pressure immediately distal to a stenosis may be lower than the pressure 2 to 3 vessel diameters downstream. This small pressure difference is called pressure recovery and is a result of the conversion of kinetic energy into pressure energy as laminar flow is restored. Although not typically seen with intermediate stenoses, pressure recovery can be avoided by advancing the transducer portion of the pressure wire at least 2 to 3 vessel diameters beyond the stenosis.

Effects of Central Venous Pressure

FFR was formally derived and validated as Pd – Pv/Pa – Pv during maximal hyperemia. In practice, the effects of central venous pressure are typically presumed to be negligible, and FFR is assumed to be approximately equal to Pd/Pa. However, in a study of 66 patients using invasive measurement of right atrial pressure (Pv) and an FFR cutoff of 0.75, Perera and colleagues[3] demonstrated that 14% of all lesions would be misclassified as insignificant when Pv was ignored. Presuming a fixed Pv value of 5, 8, or 10 mm Hg improved sensitivity but decreased specificity. In a mathematical analysis, Kumar[4] showed that (1) any elevation in Pv can only make the estimated FFR lower, so that there is no value to measuring Pa when FFR is less than or equal to 0.80, (2) the effect of Pv is less in hypertensive patients, and (3) that the use of an FFR threshold value of less than or equal to 0.80 reduced the chance of a false-negative FFR compared with a threshold of less than or equal to 0.75 (Fig. 11).

The practice of ignoring the effect of Pv has been validated by the robust clinical outcomes of the Fractional Flow Reserve to Determine Appropriateness of Angioplasty in Moderate

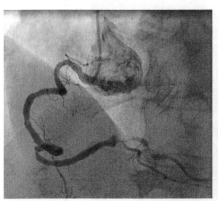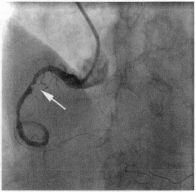

Fig. 10. Wire straightening artifact. The stiffness of the wire can straighten the tortuosity of a vessel, creating kinks in the artery (*arrow*) that may be hemodynamically significant.

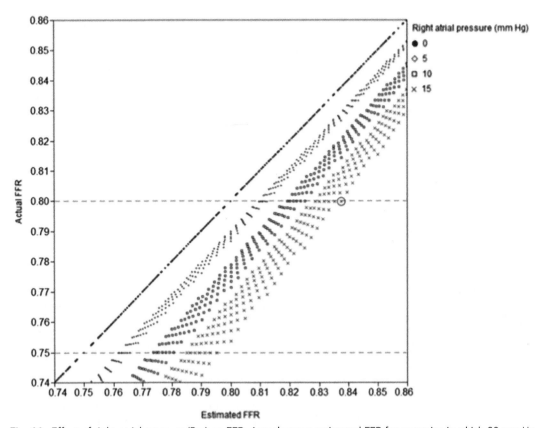

Fig. 11. Effect of right atrial pressure (Pra) on FFR. Actual versus estimated FFR for scenarios in which 80 mm Hg ≤ Pa ≤110 mm Hg showing progressive decrease in actual FFR with increasing Pra. At a Pra of 15 mm Hg, an estimated FFR of 0.838 (*circled*) corrects to 0.80. (*From* Kumar G. Letter to the editor: the influence of right atrial pressure on fractional flow reserve. J Invasive Cardiol 2012;24(10):A43; with permission.)

Coronary Stenoses (DEFER), Fractional Flow Reserve versus Angiography for Multivessel Evaluation (FAME), and FAME II trials, which did not require measurement of Pv to estimate FFR in a selected population of patients with stable angina. The use of FFR less than or equal to 0.80 rather than less than 0.75 effectively captures most patients who might have had a false-negative FFR because of elevated Pv. However, in patients with hypotension or congestive heart failure, incorporation of Pv measurements adheres more closely with the theory of FFR and may be clinically appropriate.

LIMITATIONS OF METHODS FOR INDUCTION OF HYPEREMIA
Methylxanthines and Adenosine Maximal Hyperemia
Methylxanthines such as caffeine, theobromine (from chocolate), and theophylline are competitive antagonists of the adenosine receptor. It is generally recommended that all such substances be withheld before studies using adenosine to obtain an optimal hyperemic response. However, the potency of theophylline is many times greater than that of caffeine and the clinical effect of dietary methylxanthines on FFR measurements may be modest.[5] A small 10-patient study using IV caffeine to reach clinically relevant concentrations (3.8 mg/L, equivalent to a triple espresso 1 hour before the procedure) showed that FFR measurements using IC adenosine hyperemia were not altered.[6] In contrast, Matsumoto and colleagues[7] recently found that caffeine at concentrations of 1.8 to 4.6 mg/L did seem to inhibit the effect of IV adenosine (FFR 0.813 compared with 0.779 with papaverine), although larger doses of IV adenosine (210 μg/kg/min) reduced the impact (Fig. 12). Avoidance of caffeine for several hours before a procedure may thus be advisable, but more severe restrictions are likely unnecessary.

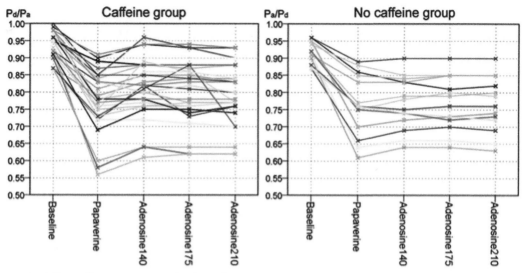

Fig. 12. Caffeine effect. FFR measured with IV adenosine at 140, 175, 210 µg/kg/min compared with papaverine in patients with and without caffeine. In patients with caffeine, FFR was overestimated with adenosine compared with papaverine. Individual values of Pd/Pa ratios at baseline and during hyperemia induced by different stimuli. (*From* Matsumoto H, Nakatsuma K, Shimada T, et al. Effect of caffeine on intravenous adenosine-induced hyperemia in fractional flow reserve measurement. J Invasive Cardiol 2014;26(11):582; with permission.)

Intracoronary Versus Intravenous Adenosine-Induced Hyperemia

A prerequisite for obtaining accurate FFR measurements is the induction of maximal hyperemia to minimize microvascular resistance. IV adenosine is widely regarded as the gold standard, although investigation into other methods of maximal hyperemia induction has been well documented. The standard doses of IC adenosine produces submaximal hyperemia relative to IV adenosine in 10% to 15% of patients, thus overestimating FFR and underestimating stenosis severity.[8] However, because of additional time and cost when giving IV adenosine, many operators prefer IC adenosine. To

compare the routes of adenosine administration, De Luca and colleagues[9] demonstrated a progressive, dose-dependent increase in the number of patients with FFR less than 0.75 with increasing IC adenosine doses up to 720 µg (Fig. 13). These data show that IC adenosine is an effective alternative to the current standard IV adenosine.[9–11]

Peripheral Versus Central Intravenous Adenosine Infusion

Controversy exists around the adequacy of adenosine infusion when given via a peripheral compared with a central vein. Based on the short half-life and intravascular deactivation of

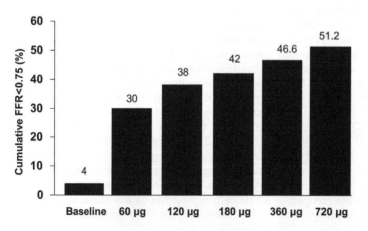

Fig. 13. Bar graph shows the cumulative percentage of patients with FFR less than or equal to 0.75 with increasing dose of adenosine. (*From* De Luca G, Venegoni L, Iorio S, et al. Effects of increasing doses of intracoronary adenosine on the assessment of fractional flow reserve. JACC Cardiovasc Interv 2011;4(10): 1083.)

adenosine, peripheral administration might result in decreased adenosine delivery. However, multiple studies using antecubital, forearm, and hand venous access sites have documented that peripheral infusion of adenosine produces comparable FFR values to central infusion.[12,13] The time to peak hyperemia for central adenosine is on an average 22 seconds faster than that for the peripheral route.[14] During peripheral IV adenosine administration, one must ensure that the blood pressure cuff is deflated or placed on the contralateral arm, so as not to interfere with the infusion. Similarly, potential venous obstructions such as pacemakers, dialysis catheters, or deep venous thrombosis may interfere with venous flow, requiring central adenosine to ensure adequate delivery.

Variable Responses to Intravenous Adenosine Infusion

Prior studies have shown FFR measurement to be largely independent of hemodynamic changes in heart rate, contractility, and blood pressure.[15,16] Theoretically, once maximal hyperemia is achieved, it can be sustained with continuous adenosine infusion, and FFR measurements should be stable enough to perform pullback measurements or multivessel assessment. However, the authors have shown that over the course of a single continuous, peripheral IV adenosine infusion, there is frequently an increase in the FFR ratio after the initial lowest Pd/Pa.[17] Among 68 patients, this increase in the Pd/Pa ratio averaged 0.08, with 28% of recordings crossing the ischemic threshold of 0.80.

Several patterns of pressure causing an FFR increase are identifiable. The most frequent pattern was that of Pd rising more than the Pa (**Fig. 14**) or fluctuating in a phasic pattern (**Fig. 15**). Using a combined pressure and flow wire, these patterns can be shown to be associated with an attenuation of the hyperemic response to continuous adenosine (**Fig. 16**), typically after 2 minutes of infusion. Matsumoto

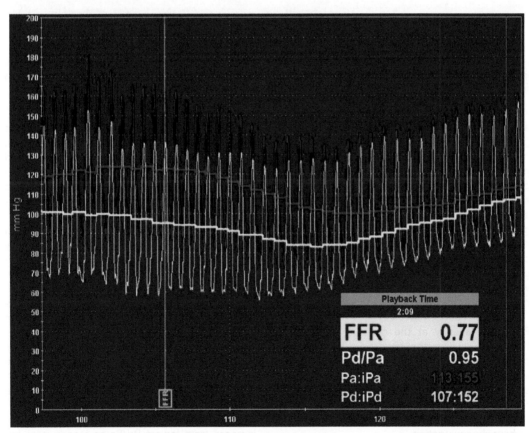

Fig. 14. Pd rising more than Pa after maximal hyperemia during continuous adenosine infusion; this may reflect attenuation of adenosine hyperemia after prolonged (>90 second) infusion. (*From* Seto AH, Tehrani DM, Bharmal MI, et al. Variations of coronary hemodynamic responses to intravenous adenosine infusion: implications for fractional flow reserve measurements. Catheter Cardiovasc Interv 2014;84(3):421; with permission.)

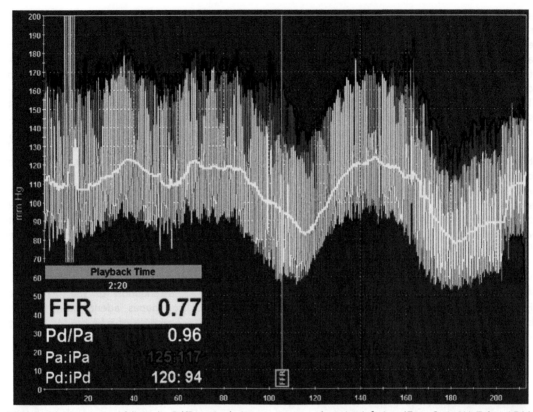

Fig. 15. Phasic rises and falls in the Pd/Pa ratio during continuous adenosine infusion. (*From* Seto AH, Tehrani DM, Bharmal MI, et al. Variations of coronary hemodynamic responses to intravenous adenosine infusion: implications for fractional flow reserve measurements. Catheter Cardiovasc Interv 2014;84(3):421; with permission.)

and colleagues[7] similarly found that a phasic pattern of FFR increase after 90 seconds occurs more frequently in patients with caffeine. It is possible that this phenomenon is due to inadequate delivery of IV adenosine, saturation of the vascular smooth muscle A_{2A} receptor, or exhaustion of cyclic AMP precursors. In a more general sense, the physiologic homeostatic response to an artificially induced coronary hyperemic and vasodilated state would be expected to be compensatory vasoconstriction, whether through adenosine receptors, mechanoreceptors, or other pathways.

A second pattern involves a sudden spike in Pa pressure early at the onset of hyperemia (Fig. 17), causing the lowest Pd/Pa value to occur before any significant drop in Pd. Given that this sudden increase in Pa was brief and often associated with symptoms, it may be due to a neurologic reflex of systemic vasoconstriction in response to the sensation of hyperemia or bronchoconstriction.[18]

The last pattern of FFR change involves a fall in Pa relative to Pd. Adenosine can cause variable degrees of systemic vasodilation in different individuals, occasionally causing more systemic than coronary vasodilation (Fig. 18). Echavarría-Pinto and colleagues[19] described such changes as being associated with a high body mass index, and possibly due to impaired coronary microcirculatory adenosine A_1 receptors.

Tarkin and colleagues[20] have demonstrated that adenosine affects systemic and coronary vascular beds differentially, even when stable hyperemia is eventually achieved. Typically, a fall in Pd occurs early at the onset of hyperemia, whereas Pa is maintained for another 5 to 10 seconds before also falling to a stable level. In practice and based on the programming of commercial FFR software, the lowest Pd/Pa values during the recording is taken as the FFR value by which clinical decisions are made. However, the FAME investigators used central adenosine infusion and measured FFR at steady-state hyperemia (after Pa has fallen). While the numerical increase from lowest Pd/Pa to steady-state hyperemic Pd/Pa has been described by the FAME investigators as 0.01 to 0.02, Tarkin and colleagues[20] found an average increase of

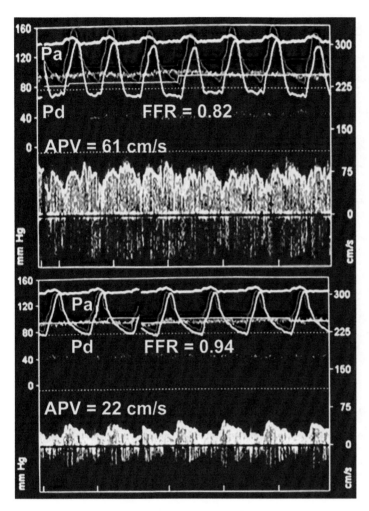

Fig. 16. Instability of hyperemic flow with prolonged adenosine infusion. A combined pressure and flow wire (ComboWire, Volcano Corp, Rancho Mirage, CA) measures an average peak velocity (APV) of 61 cm/s and an FFR value of 0.82 at maximal hyperemia (*top panel*). After continued adenosine infusion (*bottom panel*), the APV decreases to 22 cm/s and the FFR value increases to 0.94, indicating attenuation of adenosine hyperemia despite continued infusion. Phasic responses can also be demonstrated. (*From* Seto AH, Tehrani DM, Bharmal MI, et al. Variations of coronary hemodynamic responses to intravenous adenosine infusion: implications for fractional flow reserve measurements. Catheter Cardiovasc Interv 2014;84(3):422; with permission.)

0.04. As the FAME studies have demonstrated robust clinical outcomes based on FFR measured at steady-state hyperemia, the thoughtful operator should avoid revascularizing a lesion that transiently has a Pd/Pa of 0.78 to 0.79 for a few seconds early during adenosine infusion but a Pd/Pa of 0.82 at steady-state hyperemia.

In summary:

1. Dynamic and variable hemodynamic responses may occur with IV adenosine infusion.
2. If steady-state Pd/Pa values are not sustained, operators should use the lowest hyperemic Pd/Pa as the true FFR value to avoid the possibility of a false-negative FFR.
3. If steady-state hyperemia is generated, one should measure the FFR as the lowest steady-state value after initial hyperemia occurs, as initial changes may be transient.

LIMITATIONS OF A SINGLE CUTOFF VALUE

After multiple clinical trials including DEFER, FAME, and FAME II, the FFR-guided approach has been shown to be superior to the angiographic approach to revascularization. Ultimately, these studies supported FFR less than or equal to 0.80 as the threshold value for intervention.[21] However, Petraco and colleagues[22] demonstrated the limitations of any single cutoff value when the method and tools have inherent imprecision. The investigators found that in the gray area zone of 0.77 to 0.83, the chance of an FFR value crossing the threshold of 0.80 upon remeasurement of the same lesion 10 minutes later was 20%. The closer the initial FFR value was to 0.80, the higher the likelihood of crossing the threshold value. Like any diagnostic test, FFR has an inherent coefficient of variation, largely because of the variable physiologic response to adenosine.

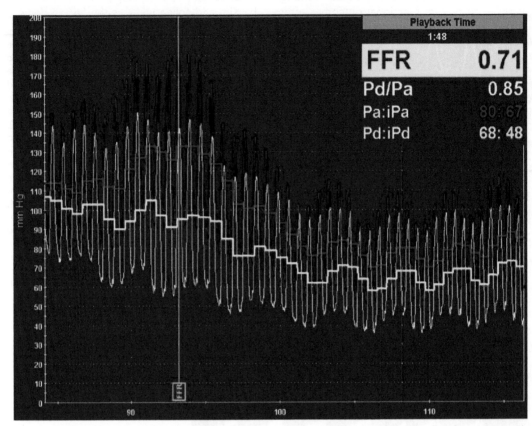

Fig. 17. Sudden spike of Pa early in the onset of hyperemia; this may reflect a neurologic reflex in response to the sensation of hyperemia. (*From* Seto AH, Tehrani DM, Bharmal MI, et al. Variations of coronary hemodynamic responses to intravenous adenosine infusion: implications for fractional flow reserve measurements. Catheter Cardiovasc Interv 2014;84(3):421; with permission.)

A more nuanced approach is suggested by a patient-level meta-analysis of all FFR trials by Johnson and colleagues.[23] The investigators found that the clinical outcome of patients was directly correlated with their FFR measurement, such that lower FFR values were associated with a higher risk of cardiovascular complications. Thus rather than a simple binary outcome, FFR provides a continuum of risk based on the severity of the ischemia that can be demonstrated. Patients with the most severe lesions would benefit most from revascularization, whereas more borderline lesions could be potentially deferred if the clinical situation suggests (ie, a higher risk of PCI complications, or minimal symptoms).

Fractional Flow Reserve in Difficult Anatomic Subsets

The measurement and interpretation of FFR is complicated by the specific coronary physiology of tandem lesions, bifurcation lesions, left main stenoses, and acute coronary syndromes (ACSs); these are dealt with elsewhere in this issue in more detail by Mallidi and Lotfi,[24] with the following being the key points:

1. The presence of tandem stenosis influences the hemodynamic significance of an individual stenosis. Revascularization of a single stenosis may cause the measured gradient of a second stenosis to increase.
2. The microvasculature is dysfunctional in ACSs. FFR of culprit vessel lesions may be associated false-negative results in the acute setting, which may become positive after myocardial flow recovers. However, if FFR is abnormal in the ACS lesion, it can be relied upon as reflective of lesion severity.
3. The presence of collaterals increases the effective myocardial bed supplied by the donor artery, with a greater degree of visual-functional mismatch, wherein the increased bed flow potentially causes even minor angiographic stenoses to be physiologically significant.

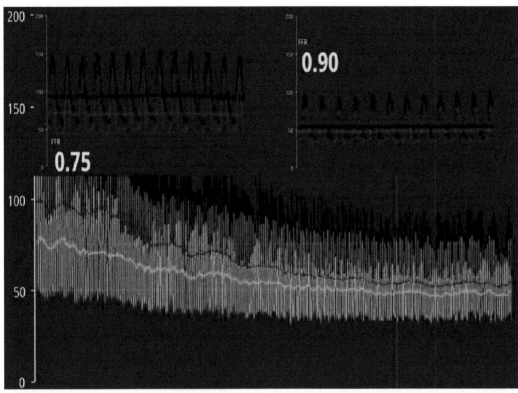

Fig. 18. Systemic hypotension, with Pa falling relative to the Pd during continuous adenosine infusion. Adenosine can cause variable degrees of systemic vasodilation in different individuals, in some cases causing more systemic than coronary vasodilation. (*From* Seto AH, Tehrani DM, Bharmal MI, et al. Variations of coronary hemodynamic responses to intravenous adenosine infusion: implications for fractional flow reserve measurements. Catheter Cardiovasc Interv 2014;84(3):421; with permission.)

SUMMARY

FFR provides a rapid, safe, and reliable technique to determine the functional significance of epicardial coronary stenoses in the catheterization laboratory. Understanding the potential technical challenges of pressure measurement and the limitations of adenosine hyperemia will prepare the operator for any unexpected findings and avoid any miscalculations.

REFERENCES

1. Pijls NH, van Son JA, Kirkeeide RL, et al. Experimental basis of determining maximum coronary, myocardial, and collateral blood flow by pressure measurements for assessing functional stenosis severity before and after percutaneous transluminal coronary angioplasty. Circulation 1993;87(4):1354–67.

2. De Bruyne B, Stockbroeckx J, Demoor D, et al. Role of side holes in guide catheters: observations on coronary pressure and flow. Cathet Cardiovasc Diagn 1994;33(2):145–52.

3. Perera D, Biggart S, Postema P, et al. Right atrial pressure: can it be ignored when calculating fractional flow reserve and collateral flow index? J Am Coll Cardiol 2004;44(10):2089–91.

4. Kumar G. Letter to the editor: the influence of right atrial pressure on fractional flow reserve. J Invasive Cardiol 2012;24(10):A43–4.

5. Salcedo J, Kern MJ. Effects of caffeine and theophylline on coronary hyperemia induced by adenosine or dipyridamole. Catheter Cardiovasc Interv 2009;74(4):598–605.

6. Aqel RA, Zoghbi GJ, Trimm JR, et al. Effect of caffeine administered intravenously on intracoronary-administered adenosine-induced coronary hemodynamics in patients with coronary artery disease. Am J Cardiol 2004;93(3):343–6.

7. Matsumoto H, Nakatsuma K, Shimada T, et al. Effect of caffeine on intravenous adenosine-induced hyperemia in fractional flow reserve measurement. J Invasive Cardiol 2014;26(11):580–5.

8. Pijls NH, Kern MJ, Yock PG, et al. Practice and potential pitfalls of coronary pressure measurement. Catheter Cardiovasc Interv 2000;49(1):1–16.

9. De Luca G, Venegoni L, Iorio S, et al. Effects of increasing doses of intracoronary adenosine on the assessment of fractional flow reserve. JACC Cardiovasc Interv 2011;4(10):1079–84.

10. Casella G, Leibig M, Schiele TM, et al. Are high doses of intracoronary adenosine an alternative to standard intravenous adenosine for the assessment of fractional flow reserve? Am Heart J 2004;148(4): 590–5.

11. Leone AM, Porto I, De Caterina AR, et al. Maximal hyperemia in the assessment of fractional flow reserve: intracoronary adenosine versus intracoronary sodium nitroprusside versus intravenous adenosine: the NASCI (Nitroprussiato versus Adenosina nelle Stenosi Coronariche Intermedie) study. JACC Cardiovasc Interv 2012;5(4):402–8.

12. Seo MK, Koo BK, Kim JH, et al. Comparison of hyperemic efficacy between central and peripheral venous adenosine infusion for fractional flow reserve measurement. Circ Cardiovasc Interv 2012;5(3):401–5.

13. Lindstaedt M, Bojara W, Holland-Letz T, et al. Adenosine-induced maximal coronary hyperemia for myocardial fractional flow reserve measurements: comparison of administration by femoral venous versus antecubital venous access. Clin Res Cardiol 2009;98(11):717–23.

14. Scott P, Sirker A, Dworakowski R, et al. FFR in the transradial era - can we leave femoral out of it? A comparative study of the extent, rapidity and stability of hyperemia from hand and femoral venous routes of adenosine administration. JACC Cardiovasc Interv 2015;8:527–35.

15. Pijls NH, Van Gelder B, Van der Voort P, et al. Fractional flow reserve. A useful index to evaluate the influence of an epicardial coronary stenosis on myocardial blood flow. Circulation 1995;92(11):3183–93.

16. de Bruyne B, Bartunek J, Sys SU, et al. Simultaneous coronary pressure and flow velocity measurements in humans. Feasibility, reproducibility, and hemodynamic dependence of coronary flow velocity reserve, hyperemic flow versus pressure slope index, and fractional flow reserve. Circulation 1996;94(8):1842–9.

17. Seto AH, Tehrani DM, Bharmal MI, et al. Variations of coronary hemodynamic responses to intravenous adenosine infusion: implications for fractional flow reserve measurements. Catheter Cardiovasc Interv 2014;84(3):416–25.

18. Biaggioni I. Contrasting excitatory and inhibitory effects of adenosine in blood pressure regulation. Hypertension 1992;20(4):457–65.

19. Echavarría-Pinto M, Gonzalo N, Ibanez B, et al. Low coronary microcirculatory resistance associated with profound hypotension during intravenous adenosine infusion: implications for the functional assessment of coronary stenoses. Circ Cardiovasc Interv 2014;7(1):35–42.

20. Tarkin JM, Nijjer S, Sen S, et al. Hemodynamic response to intravenous adenosine and its effect on fractional flow reserve assessment: results of the Adenosine for the Functional Evaluation of Coronary Stenosis Severity (AFFECTS) study. Circ Cardiovasc Interv 2013;6(6):654–61.

21. De Bruyne B, Pijls NH, Kalesan B, et al. Fractional flow reserve-guided PCI versus medical therapy in stable coronary disease. N Engl J Med 2012; 367(11):991–1001.

22. Petraco R, Sen S, Nijjer S, et al. Fractional flow reserve-guided revascularization: practical implications of a diagnostic gray zone and measurement variability on clinical decisions. JACC Cardiovasc Interv 2013;6(3):222–5.

23. Johnson NP, Toth GG, Lai D, et al. Prognostic value of fractional flow reserve: linking physiologic severity to clinical outcomes. J Am Coll Cardiol 2014;64(16):1641–54.

24. Mallidi J, Lotfi. Fractional Flow Reserve for the Evaluation of Tandem and Bifurcation Lesions, Left Main, and Acute Coronary Syndromes. Intervent Cardiol Clin 2015, in press.

Landmark Fractional Flow Reserve Trials

Donald R. Lynch Jr, MD, William F. Fearon, MD*

KEYWORDS

- Coronary artery disease • Coronary ischemia • Coronary physiology • Fractional flow reserve
- Percutaneous coronary intervention

KEY POINTS

- Fractional flow reserve (FFR) has been validated using a true gold standard for noninvasive ischemia (a combination of 3 stress test modalities).
- The Fractional Flow Reserve to Determine Appropriateness of Angioplasty in Moderate Coronary Stenoses (DEFER) trial established the ability of FFR to identify intermediate lesions in which revascularization can safely be deferred.
- The Fractional Flow Reserve versus Angiography for Multivessel Evaluation (FAME) trial demonstrated the safety and feasibility of FFR-guided revascularization in stable and unstable patients with multivessel coronary disease.
- FAME 2 trial demonstrated higher rates of urgent revascularization, myocardial infarction (MI), and death in patients with stable angina (SA) who have functionally significant lesions based on FFR, which are treated with medical therapy.
- FFR has been shown to be cost effective through reduction in the number of unnecessary stents and reduction in adverse cardiac events.

INTRODUCTION

Historically, the gold standard for assessment of coronary disease was based on visual estimation of angiographic stenosis. The anatomic lumenogram information provided by coronary angiography is limited in its ability to assess physiologic significance of identified lesions and their likelihood of causing coronary ischemia. The clinical significance of a coronary lesion depends on the extent of viable myocardium supplied by the vessel. Approximately 39% of angiographically obstructive coronary stenoses have no functional significance.[1] Revascularization of nonhemodynamically significant coronary lesions may lead to worse clinical outcomes.

Several strategies have been used to identify and localize coronary ischemia. Noninvasive stress testing has been used as a first-line modality for diagnosis and risk stratification of patients with known or suspected coronary disease. Noninvasive techniques are useful from a population standpoint and have been implemented in appropriateness guidelines.[2] However, each of these imaging methods has limited spatial resolution and diagnostic accuracy, particularly in patients with multivessel coronary disease.[3] As shown in Fig. 1, myocardial perfusion imaging with single-photon emission computed tomography has poor correlation with FFR among patients with multivessel disease.[4]

Functional lesion testing using FFR has been validated in the assessment of intermediate coronary stenosis. FFR uses a coronary wire equipped with a miniaturized pressure transducer to measure the ratio of distal coronary pressure, distal to a coronary stenosis, to the proximal pressure during maximal coronary vasodilation.[5] Unlike coronary flow reserve, FFR is independent of variation in hemodynamic parameters,

---

Division of Cardiovascular Medicine, Stanford University Medical Center, Stanford University School of Medicine, Stanford, CA, USA
* Corresponding author. Stanford University Medical Center, 300 Pasteur Drive, H2103, Stanford, CA 94305.
E-mail address: wfearon@stanford.edu

Intervent Cardiol Clin 4 (2015) 435–441
http://dx.doi.org/10.1016/j.iccl.2015.06.004
2211-7458/15/$ – see front matter © 2015 Elsevier Inc. All rights reserved.

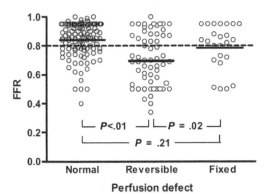

Fig. 1. Correlation of FFR and type of defect detected by myocardial perfusion imaging. (*From* Melikian N, De Bondt P, Tonino P, et al. Fractional flow reserve and myocardial perfusion imaging in patients with angiographic multivessel coronary artery disease. JACC Cardiovasc Interv 2010;3:311.)

such as heart rate, systemic blood pressure, and stroke volume. Importantly, FFR allows on-the-table hemodynamic assessment of coronary lesions overcoming many of the limitations of noninvasive evaluation modalities. An FFR value less than or equal to 0.80 has been validated for identification of ischemic lesions. Importantly, lesions with an FFR of greater than 0.80 can be managed safely without revascularization. Recent trials have demonstrated the superiority of FFR-based revascularization strategies over traditional angiography-guided revascularization. Herein, the authors review the landmark trials that validated FFR and its role in revascularization decisions.

VALIDATION IN COMPARISON TO NONINVASIVE ISCHEMIA ASSESSMENT

Pijls and colleagues[6] correlated FFR values with results of noninvasive stress test modalities (bicycle exercise testing, thallium scintigraphy, and stress echocardiography) among 45 patients presenting with chest pain and found to have moderate coronary lesions. Although there was no true gold standard for assessment of myocardial ischemia, the researchers used the combination of results of the 3 stress test modalities to establish a true noninvasive standard. The accuracy of any one stress test is 70% to 80%; however, the use of the combination of 3 test increases the accuracy to greater than 95% using Bayes theorem. Among the 21 patients with an FFR less than 0.75, myocardial ischemia was demonstrated on at least one of the stress tests. Following revascularization, the FFR values normalized. Among 21 of the 24 patients with FFR values greater than or

equal to 0.75, there was no evidence of myocardial ischemia on any of the 3 stress test modalities. These patients were ultimately followed up for 14 months and remained free of revascularization during this time. Using a cutoff value of 0.75 for diagnosis of myocardial ischemia, this study demonstrated a sensitivity of 88% and specificity of 100% for FFR. This study also established early safety of deferral of revascularization for moderate coronary lesions with FFR values greater than or equal to 0.75.

SAFETY OF REVASCULARIZATION DEFERRAL WITH NORMAL FRACTIONAL FLOW RESERVE IN SINGLE-VESSEL CORONARY DISEASE

The long-term safety of deferring percutaneous revascularization of moderate coronary lesions with FFR values greater than or equal to 0.75 was subsequently demonstrated in the DEFER trial.[7] A total of 325 patients referred for elective percutaneous intervention of moderate de novo coronary lesions (defined as >50% diameter stenosis) with no documented myocardial ischemia within the prior 2 months were randomized to one of 2 groups based on the FFR value. All patients with FFR less than 0.75 underwent percutaneous transluminal coronary angioplasty (PTCA) as planned (reference group, n = 144). If the FFR was greater than or equal to 0.75, patients were randomized to either deferral of intervention (n = 91) or performance of PTCA as planned (n = 90). Among patients in the deferral and performance groups, event-free survival was similar at 24 months (89% vs 83%, P = .27). In contrast, patients in the reference group had a significantly lower event-free survival at 12 and 24 months of 80% and 78%, respectively, likely due to a greater burden of atherosclerosis. The proportion of patients with angina-free survival was similar between the deferral and PTCA groups at 1 year but was significantly higher among patients in the deferral group at 24 months (70% vs 51%, P = .02). This pivotal randomized trial established the short-term safety of deferring intervention for angiographically moderate lesions with nonischemic FFR values.

In a follow-up study from the DEFER trial,[8] event-free survival out to 5 years was not significantly different between the deferral and performance groups (80% vs 73%; P = .52). The combined rate of cardiac death and acute myocardial infarction (AMI) was 3.3% and 7.9% in the deferral and performance groups, respectively (P = .21), as shown in **Figs. 2** and **3**.

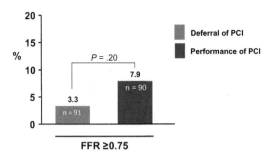

Fig. 2. Cardiac death and MI rates during 5-year follow-up of patients in deferral and performance groups of DEFER cohort. PCI, percutaneous coronary intervention. (*From* Pijls NH, van Schaardenburgh P, Manoharan G, et al. Percutaneous coronary intervention of functionally nonsignificant stenosis: 5-year follow-up of the DEFER study. J Am Coll Cardiol 2007;49:2109.)

Among patients with a functionally nonsignificant stenosis by FFR, the overall rate of death or acute myocardial infarct was less than 1% per year when managed medically; this rate was not changed by percutaneous intervention. There was significant improvement in angina status in all 3 groups at 2- and 5-year follow-ups in comparison to time of index procedure. This effect was most prominent among patients in the reference group, who had FFR less than 0.75, validating the long-term clinical benefit of revascularization of hemodynamically significant lesions at 5 years ($P = .028$). Collectively, these findings demonstrate the long-term benefit of FFR-guided revascularization of angiographically moderate lesions. Importantly, there was a trend toward increased rates of death and AMI among

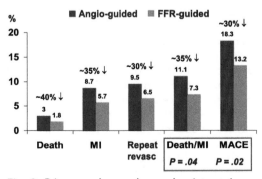

Fig. 3. Primary and secondary end points at 1 year among patients randomized to angiography-guided versus FFR-guided PCI. MACE, major adverse cardiac events; Revasc, revascularization. (*Adapted from* Tonino PA, De Bruyne B, Pijls NH, et al. Fractional flow reserve versus angiography for guiding percutaneous coronary intervention. N Engl J Med 2009;360:213–24.)

patients with functionally insignificant lesions who underwent revascularization.

FRACTIONAL-FLOW-RESERVE-GUIDED REVASCULARIZATION IN MULTIVESSEL DISEASE

While prior studies demonstrated the safety of FFR-guided single vessel revascularization, the large randomized multicenter FAME trial[9] evaluated whether routine FFR-guided intervention with drug-eluting stents improved outcome compared with angiography alone. A total of 1005 patients presenting with both stable and unstable coronary disease who were found to have multivessel disease (defined as coronary artery stenoses of at least 50% of vessel diameter in at least 2 major epicardial coronary arteries) were enrolled. Patients were excluded if less than 5 days had elapsed after ST-segment elevation myocardial infarction, if there was non-ST-segment elevation myocardial infarction (NSTEMI) with creatine kinase levels greater than 1000 U/L, and if they had angiographically significant left main coronary artery disease, previous coronary artery bypass, cardiogenic shock, extremely tortuous or calcified coronary arteries, life expectancy less than 2 years, or contraindication to placement of drug-eluting stents. Percutaneous intervention was performed in the FFR-guided percutaneous coronary intervention (PCI) group if the measured value was less than or equal to 0.80. The average number of angiographically significant lesions per patient was not significantly different between the FFR-guided (N = 509) and angiography-alone groups (N = 496) (2.7 vs 2.8; $P = .34$); however, the FFR-guided PCI group received significantly fewer stents per patient (1.9 vs 2.7; $P<.001$). There was a significant reduction in the composite primary outcome of death, MI, and repeat revascularization at 1 year among patients in the FFR-guided group compared with those in the angiography-alone group (13.2% vs 18.3%; $P = .02$) Fig. 2. The combined secondary end point of death or MI at 1 year was significantly lower in the FFR-guided group (7.3% vs 11.1%; $P = .04$). The percentage of patients with angina-free survival at 1 year was not significantly different between the FFR-guided and angiography-alone groups (81% vs 78%; $P = .20$). Procedural time was similar between the FFR-guided and angiography-alone groups (71 vs 70 minutes; $P = .51$); however, the amount of contrast used was significantly less for the FFR-guided group (272 vs 302 mL; $P<.001$). The mean index procedural cost was significantly lower for patients in the FFR-guided group ($5332 vs $6007 P<.002). The length of hospital stay for index procedure was similar between the groups. In the FAME trial, FFR guidance allowed more judicious application of PCI while still achieving a functionally complete revascularization. The avoidance of unnecessary stents decreased both periprocedural events and late stent-related complications, resulting in improved outcomes in the FFR-guided group. In a formal cost-effectiveness evaluation, the FFR-guided approach to PCI was found to be a dominant strategy, one of those unique technologies that is cost saving, not only improving outcomes but also saving money.[10] In summary, this study demonstrated the feasibility, cost-effectiveness, and short-term safety of FFR-guided PCI among both stable and unstable patients with multivessel disease.

At 2-year follow-up, the composite rate of mortality or MI remained significantly lower in the FFR-guided PCI group compared with the angiography group (8.4 vs 12.9%; $P = .02$).[11] The revascularization rate at 2 years was similar in FFR- and angiography-guided groups (10.6% vs 12.7%; $P = .30$). There was a trend toward reduction in major adverse cardiac events (MACE) among patients in the FFR group compared with those in the angiography group (17.9% vs 22.4%; $P = .08$). Angina-free survival continued to be similar between the 2 groups at 2-year follow-up. Among patients in the FFR-guided group, there were 9 (1.6%) late MIs, which could potentially be due to one of the 513 deferred lesions in these patients. However, 8 of these were related to a previously placed stent or a new coronary lesion, meaning that the rate of MI at 2 years in deferred lesions was 0.2%. Exactly 10.4% of patients in the FFR-guided PCI group required repeat revascularization; however, 7.2% of these were related to restenosis or a new lesion, translating to a rate of revascularization for deferred lesions of 3.2%. These results confirmed the continued efficacy of FFR-guided PCI among patients with multivessel disease at 2-year follow-up.

A subsequent analysis of patients within the FFR-guided arm of the FAME trial[1] evaluated the accuracy of visual angiographic characterization of lesion severity, illustrated in Fig. 4. Before randomization into the FAME trial, operators categorized significant lesions based on visual diameter stenosis as 50% to 70%, 71% to 90%, and 91% to 100%. Of lesions graded as 50% to 70%, approximately 35% were functionally significant by FFR. Only 80% of lesions rated as 71% to 90% were significant by FFR, and 96%

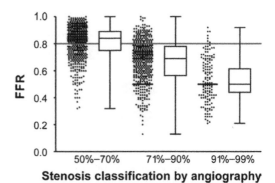

Fig. 4. Angiographic lesion characterization (50%–70%, 71%–90%, and 91%–99%) and FFR values. The horizontal line denotes FFR cutoff of 0.80 for myocardial ischemia. (*From* Tonino PA, Fearon WF, De Bruyne B, et al. Angiographic versus functional severity of coronary artery stenoses in the FAME study fractional flow reserve versus angiography in multivessel evaluation. J Am Coll Cardiol 2010;55:2818.)

of the lesions characterized as 91% to 100% were functionally significant. These results highlight the high rate of functionally insignificant lesions despite angiographic appearance.

The safety of FFR-guided intervention among 328 FAME patients presenting with unstable angina (UA) or NSTEMI was reported in a subanalysis of 150 subjects randomized to FFR-guided intervention and 178 subjects randomized to angiography.[12] Patients presenting with UA/NSTEMI compared with SA had a significantly higher rate of the combined outcome of death, MI, and repeated revascularization at 2 years (24.1% vs 18.2%; $P = .03$). There was also a significantly higher incidence of the composite of death or MI (13.7% vs 9.2%; $P = .04$). The use of FFR-guided intervention among patients presenting with UA/NSTEMI compared with SA resulted in a similar reduction in risk of major adverse events at 2 years (Absolute Risk Reduction [ARR] 3.7% vs 5.1%; P 0.92). Similar to the overall cohort, patients with UA/NSTEMI randomized to FFR-guided PCI compared with angiography received significantly less stents (1.9 vs 2.9; $P<.01$) and had less contrast use (269 mL vs 308 mL; $P = .01$). These results suggest that patients presenting with acute coronary syndrome without ST elevation experience similar beneficial effects of FFR-guided PCI.

The SYNTAX (SYNergy between PCI with TAXUS and Cardiac Surgery) score is an angiography-based calculation incorporating lesion characteristics for prediction of clinical outcome following PCI among patients with multivessel or left main disease.[13] Reclassification of patients with a functional SYNTAX score (FSS) by incorporating FFR lesion assessment resulted in a better predictive accuracy for MACE at 1 year (Harrell's C 0.677 vs 0.630; $P = .002$).[14] The FSS counts only lesions that are functionally significant with FFR less than or equal to 0.80. Applying the FSS to the classic SYNTAX score moved approximately 32% of patients into a lower risk group. MACE at 1 year for patients in the low-, medium-, and high-FSS groups were significantly different (9.0%, 11.3%, and 26.7%, respectively), as can be seen in **Fig. 5**. In a multivariate analysis, only procedure time and FSS were independent predictors of 1-year MACE. These results suggest enhanced outcome prediction using the FSS.

FRACTIONAL-FLOW-RESERVE-GUIDED REVASCULARIZATION AMONG PATIENTS WITH STABLE CORONARY DISEASE

Among patients with SA for which PCI is considered, FFR-guided revascularization was recently evaluated against optimal medical therapy in the FAME 2 trial.[15] All patients who had SA and at least 1 angiographically significant stenosis (>50% narrowed) in a major epicardial artery were eligible for the study. FFR was measured in all diseased vessels, and if there was at least 1 functionally significant stenosis (FFR $\leq$0.80), the patient was randomized to either FFR-guided PCI with optimal medical therapy or to optimal medical therapy alone. The goal was to randomize approximately 1600 patients with the primary end point being the composite of death, MI, and hospitalization requiring urgent revascularization during 2 years of follow-up. Because of a significantly higher incidence of the primary composite outcome among patients in the medical group (12.7% vs 4.3%; 95% confidence interval [CI], 0.19–0.53; $P<.001$), the independent data and safety monitoring board made the strong

recommendation to stop the trial early after the recruitment of 1220 patients. Of these 1220 patients, 880 were randomized and the remaining one-fourth of patients were found to have no functionally significant stenoses (all FFR >0.80) despite their angiographic appearance; these patients were followed up in a registry arm. The difference in the primary end point was driven primarily by a significantly higher rate of urgent revascularization among patients in the medical group (11.1% vs 1.6%; 95% CI, 0.06–0.30). There was no significant difference in the rate of death or MI. Among the registry cohort of patients (FFR $\geq$0.80), the rate of the composite outcome was 3% at a mean follow-up of 206 days, despite a similar burden of coronary disease. These results point to an increased risk of adverse cardiac events when deferring PCI of hemodynamically significant lesions; they further solidify the safety of treating hemodynamically insignificant lesions medically. However, there was significant criticism of the trial because of early halting of enrollment, which was driven primarily by the end point of urgent revascularization.

Recently, De Bruyne and colleagues[16] reported the full 2-year follow-up for FAME 2 trial participants, as illustrated in **Fig. 6**. The rate of the composite primary outcome was significantly lower among the FFR-guided revascularization group (8.7 vs 19.5%; 95% CI, 0.26–0.57). As reported previously, this was driven primarily by a reduction in rates of urgent revascularization within the PCI group (4.0 vs 16.3%; 95% CI, 0.14–0.38). Urgent revascularization prompted by MI or ischemic electrocardiographic changes were significantly more frequent within the medical therapy group (7.0% vs 3.4%, $P = .01$). After exclusion of periprocedural events within the first 1 week, the rate of death or MI was significantly lower in the PCI group (4.6% vs 8.0%; $P = .04$). This finding is particularly relevant

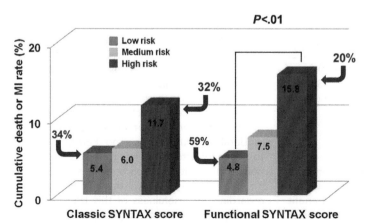

P<.01

Classic SYNTAX score   Functional SYNTAX score

Cumulative death or MI rate (%)

Low risk / Medium risk / High risk

34% / 32% / 59% / 20%

5.4 / 6.0 / 11.7 / 4.8 / 7.5 / 15.8

Fig. 5. The rates of MACE corresponding to the tertiles of SYNTAX score and functional SYNTAX score. (*From* Nam CW, Mangiacapra F, Entjes R, et al. Functional SYNTAX score for risk assessment in multivessel coronary artery disease. J Am Coll Cardiol 2011;58:1216.)

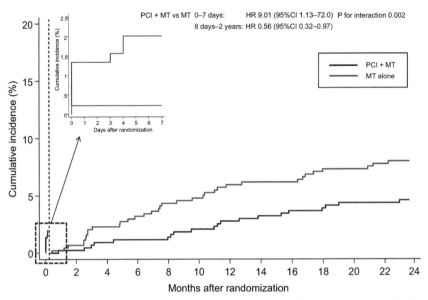

Fig. 6. Kaplan-Meier analysis for primary end point (a composite of death from any cause, nonfatal MI, or urgent revascularization) stratified on the basis of a landmark point at 7 days after randomization. HR, hazard ratio; MT, medical therapy. (*From* De Bruyne B, Fearon WF, Pijls NH, et al. Fractional flow reserve-guided PCI for stable coronary artery disease. N Engl J Med 2014;371:1212; with permission.)

because previous studies have shown that periprocedural MI is generally not prognostically important, whereas spontaneously occurring MI is a predictor of long-term mortality.[17,18] Collectively, FAME 2 suggests that FFR-guided intervention among patients with SA significantly reduces the rate of major cardiac events.

The cost-effectiveness of FFR-guided percutaneous intervention in the FAME 2 trial was recently reported.[19] Among patients with functionally significant coronary disease, baseline costs were significantly more for PCI than for medical therapy ($9927 vs $3995; P<.001). Over the ensuing year, however, this difference narrowed to $2883, because of the need for urgent revascularization and other adverse events among the medical group. Quality of life, measured with EQ-5D, was significantly improved with PCI compared with medical therapy (0.054 vs 0.001 units; P<.001). Overall, FFR-guided PCI among patients with SA provided a favorable incremental cost-effectiveness ratio of $36,000 per quality-adjusted life-year. This finding was robust on sensitivity analysis.

SUMMARY/DISCUSSION

The 3 large, multicenter, international, randomized studies reviewed[7,9,15] along with multiple registries[20,21] demonstrate the clinical benefit of FFR-guided PCI compared with angiography-guided PCI and medical therapy in a variety of patient subsets. Improved lesion characterization using FFR provides incremental value in assessment of lesion significance over conventional coronary angiography. Detection of myocardial ischemia using FFR has been shown to be comparable if not better than noninvasive stress testing while providing better localization of ischemia-producing disease among patients with multivessel disease; this has afforded improved outcomes in patients with coronary disease through revascularization of only functionally significant lesions and medical treatment of nonsignificant ones (ie, functionally complete revascularization). Among patients with SA, FFR facilitates recognition of hemodynamically significant lesions that are not optimally treated with medical therapy alone.

In summary, FFR has been shown to be superior to angiography alone in the identification and localization of lesions contributing to myocardial ischemia. FFR is superior to other existing methods in this regard and has been shown to be cost effective through reduction of adverse events. Another large, multicenter, randomized study comparing FFR-guided PCI to coronary artery bypass graft surgery in patients with multivessel coronary disease (FAME 3[22]) is underway and will provide further data regarding the usefulness of this transformative technique in our most complex patient subset.

REFERENCES

1. Tonino PA, Fearon WF, De Bruyne B, et al. Angiographic versus functional severity of coronary artery stenoses in the FAME study fractional flow reserve versus angiography in multivessel evaluation. J Am Coll Cardiol 2010;55:2816–21.

2. Patel MR, Dehmer GJ, Hirshfeld JW, et al. ACCF/SCAI/STS/AATS/AHA/ASNC/HFSA/SCCT 2012 Appropriate use criteria for coronary revascularization focused update: a report of the American College of Cardiology Foundation Appropriate Use Criteria Task Force, Society for Cardiovascular Angiography and Interventions, Society of Thoracic Surgeons, American Association for Thoracic Surgery, American Heart Association, American Society of Nuclear Cardiology, and the Society of Cardiovascular Computed Tomography. J Am Coll Cardiol 2012;59:857–81.

3. Beller GA, Ragosta M. Decision making in multivessel coronary disease: the need for physiological lesion assessment. JACC Cardiovasc Interv 2010;3:315–7.

4. Melikian N, De Bondt P, Tonino P, et al. Fractional flow reserve and myocardial perfusion imaging in patients with angiographic multivessel coronary artery disease. JACC Cardiovasc Interv 2010;3:307–14.

5. Pijls NH, van Son JA, Kirkeeide RL, et al. Experimental basis of determining maximum coronary, myocardial, and collateral blood flow by pressure measurements for assessing functional stenosis severity before and after percutaneous transluminal coronary angioplasty. Circulation 1993;87:1354–67.

6. Pijls NH, De Bruyne B, Peels K, et al. Measurement of fractional flow reserve to assess the functional severity of coronary-artery stenoses. N Engl J Med 1996;334:1703–8.

7. Bech GJ, De Bruyne B, Pijls NH, et al. Fractional flow reserve to determine the appropriateness of angioplasty in moderate coronary stenosis: a randomized trial. Circulation 2001;103:2928–34.

8. Pijls NH, van Schaardenburgh P, Manoharan G, et al. Percutaneous coronary intervention of functionally nonsignificant stenosis: 5-year follow-up of the DEFER Study. J Am Coll Cardiol 2007;49:2105–11.

9. Tonino PA, De Bruyne B, Pijls NH, et al. Fractional flow reserve versus angiography for guiding percutaneous coronary intervention. N Engl J Med 2009;360:213–24.

10. Fearon WF, Bornschein B, Tonino PA, et al. Economic evaluation of fractional flow reserve-guided percutaneous coronary intervention in patients with multivessel disease. Circulation 2010;122:2545–50.

11. Pijls NH, Fearon WF, Tonino PA, et al. Fractional flow reserve versus angiography for guiding percutaneous coronary intervention in patients with multivessel coronary artery disease: 2-year follow-up of the FAME (Fractional Flow Reserve Versus Angiography for Multivessel Evaluation) study. J Am Coll Cardiol 2010;56:177–84.

12. Sels JW, Tonino PA, Siebert U, et al. Fractional flow reserve in unstable angina and non-ST-segment elevation myocardial infarction experience from the FAME (Fractional flow reserve versus Angiography for Multivessel Evaluation) study. JACC Cardiovasc Interv 2011;4:1183–9.

13. Serruys PW, Morice MC, Kappetein AP, et al. Percutaneous coronary intervention versus coronary-artery bypass grafting for severe coronary artery disease. N Engl J Med 2009;360:961–72.

14. Nam CW, Mangiacapra F, Entjes R, et al. Functional SYNTAX score for risk assessment in multivessel coronary artery disease. J Am Coll Cardiol 2011;58:1211–8.

15. De Bruyne B, Pijls NH, Kalesan B, et al. Fractional flow reserve-guided PCI versus medical therapy in stable coronary disease. N Engl J Med 2012;367:991–1001.

16. De Bruyne B, Fearon WF, Pijls NH, et al. Fractional flow reserve-guided PCI for stable coronary artery disease. N Engl J Med 2014;371:1208–17.

17. Prasad A, Gersh BJ, Bertrand ME, et al. Prognostic significance of periprocedural versus spontaneously occurring myocardial infarction after percutaneous coronary intervention in patients with acute coronary syndromes: an analysis from the ACUITY (Acute Catheterization and Urgent Intervention Triage Strategy) trial. J Am Coll Cardiol 2009;54:477–86.

18. Damman P, Wallentin L, Fox KA, et al. Long-term cardiovascular mortality after procedure-related or spontaneous myocardial infarction in patients with non-ST-segment elevation acute coronary syndrome: a collaborative analysis of individual patient data from the FRISC II, ICTUS, and RITA-3 trials (FIR). Circulation 2012;125:568–76.

19. Fearon WF, Shilane D, Pijls NH, et al. Cost-effectiveness of percutaneous coronary intervention in patients with stable coronary artery disease and abnormal fractional flow reserve. Circulation 2013;128:1335–40.

20. Li J, Elrashidi MY, Flammer AJ, et al. Long-term outcomes of fractional flow reserve-guided vs. angiography-guided percutaneous coronary intervention in contemporary practice. Eur Heart J 2013;34:1375–83.

21. Park SJ, Ahn JM, Park GM, et al. Trends in the outcomes of percutaneous coronary intervention with the routine incorporation of fractional flow reserve in real practice. Eur Heart J 2013;34:3353–61.

22. A Comparison of Fractional Flow Reserve-Guided Percutaneous Coronary Intervention and Coronary Artery Bypass Graft Surgery in Patients with Multivessel Coronary Artery Disease (FAME 3). 2014. Available at: http://clinicaltrials.gov/show/NCT02100722. Accessed November 10, 2014.

Evaluation of Microvascular Disease and Clinical Outcomes

Christopher J. Broyd, PhD, MBBS,
Mauro Echavarria-Pinto, MD, Enrico Cerrato, MD,
Javier Escaned, MD, PhD*

KEYWORDS

- Microvasculature • Intravascular • Physiology • Outcomes

KEY POINTS

- Myocardial blood supply is controlled through an interplay of metabolic, myogenic, endothelial, and neural factors; all of which may be involved in its dysfunction.
- Intravascular physiology allows the exploration of the microvascular domain in heart disease and has the potential to obtain information with prognostic relevance.
- Because interrogation of the microvasculature using intravascular techniques allows real-time assessment, it can potentially guide intracoronary adjuvant therapy, particularly during acute coronary syndromes.
- Most intravascular microcirculatory assessment tools are based on measures of coronary flow, either alone (resting flow profile) or in combination with pressure during rest (wave intensity analysis) or hyperemia to provide downstream information.
- The selection of a method to interrogate the coronary microcirculation should be based on the suspected dominant cause of dysfunction.

INTRODUCTION

Unlike the large capacitance vessels of the epicardium, the microcirculation has a highly dynamic role in coronary blood flow and is regulated through metabolic, myogenic, endothelial, and neural influences to provide the dominant component of coronary resistance.[1,2] Microcirculatory abnormalities can arise through any of these pathways, either alone or in combination, and may convey an adverse prognosis equivalent to frank obstructive epicardial vessel disease. In addition to such marked complexity in its physiologic organization and pathophysiologic potential, it anatomically consists of vessels that are less than 300 μm in diameter that escape the spatial resolution available at coronary angiography. Therefore, although assessment of the microcirculation is essential for modern cardiologic practice, it requires tools that are both sophisticated and dynamic even though they are unable to operate with direct visualization.

At present, the most widely used intravascular investigative technique is fractional flow reserve (FFR). Although this is an excellent tool for the assessment of epicardial stenosis, it is unable to provide information on the microcirculation and, therefore, cannot offer a complete cardiac assessment of the patient in the catheter laboratory. If concomitant microvascular disease could also be quantified, a more satisfactory clinical picture could be established, which would not only aid with diagnoses but also guide immediate changes in treatment and provide an individually tailored approach.

Cardiovascular Institute, Hospital Clínico San Carlos, Madrid 28040, Spain
* Corresponding author.
E-mail address: escaned@secardiologia.es

Intervent Cardiol Clin 4 (2015) 443–457
http://dx.doi.org/10.1016/j.iccl.2015.06.005
2211-7458/15/$ – see front matter © 2015 Elsevier Inc. All rights reserved.

Additionally, although in stable patients it is possible to gain some of this additional information through other investigative modalities performed at a separate time, situations in which time is a determinant of prognosis implementation of ad hoc therapy (eg, intracoronary pharmacotherapy or thrombus aspiration during ST-elevation myocardial infarction [STEMI]) requires immediate microcirculatory quantification. A periprocedural intravascular assessment technique is optimal in this setting because results can be acted on during this short therapeutic window.

Important in the treatment of microvascular dysfunction is that this may result from several potential mechanisms, including endothelial abnormalities, arteriolar or capillary remodeling, and extravascular compression. At present, there are several methods that allow such intravascular quantification of the microvasculature, each with specific advantages for exploring these respective domains (Fig. 1). This article highlights these techniques along with the prognostic information provided by these modalities.

DIRECT ANGIOGRAPHIC ASSESSMENT

The first attempts to obtain information on the microvasculature at the time of angiography began with quantification of the radiographic density of dye as it passed through the coronary system using digital extraction technology to map its timing. This predicted the resting flow rate reasonably well and recognized an

impairment of coronary flow reserve (CFR) in patients with significant coronary stenosis[3] (Fig. 2).

The investigators of the Thrombolysis in Myocardial Infarction (TIMI) trials introduced several methods to objectively stratify coronary blood flow and thus assess microvascular health. The thrombolysis in myocardial infarction (TIMI)-flow grade is a qualitative assessment that uses contrast injected into the artery of interest and correlating it with resting flow rates from Doppler-flow wires.[4] It is relatively specific, with only TIMI-flow grade 3 displaying a normal underlying blood velocity. As such, the TIMI-flow grade after a treated myocardial infarction is correlated with outcome[5] and TIMI grade 2 has been associated with an outcome similar to that of an occluded artery.[6]

TIMI 0: Absence of complete antegrade flow

TIMI 1: Faint antegrade flow beyond the occlusion, incomplete filling of the distal coronary bed

TIMI 2: Partial reperfusion, delayed antegrade flow but with complete filling of the distal territory

TIMI 3: Normal flow, the distal coronary bed is completely filled

---

A more quantitative assessment is provided by the TIMI frame count (TFC), defined as the number of cine frames required for radiographic

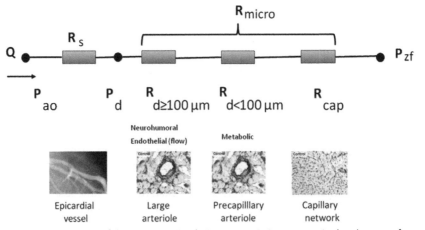

Fig. 1. Schematic representation of the coronary circulation as a resistive system. In the absence of a coronary stenosis, arteriolar tone constitutes the main seat of coronary resistance and is controlled by metabollic, myogenic, llow-dependent (enothelial) and neurogenic mechanisms. Microcirculatory dysfuntion may result from structural remodelling of arterioles or capillaries (rarefaction), dysregulation (paradoxical arteriolar vasoconstriction), hypersensitivity to vasoactive factor or adrenergic stimulation, and extravascular compression of collapsable vascular elements (capillaries). Pao, aortic pressure; Pd, pressure distal to the stenosis; Pzf, zero flow pressure; Q, coronary flow; Rcap, capillary resistance; Rmicro, microcirculatory resistance; Rd≥100mcm and Rd<100mcm, resistance of arterioles with diameters above and below 100mcm, respectively; Rs, stenosis resistance.

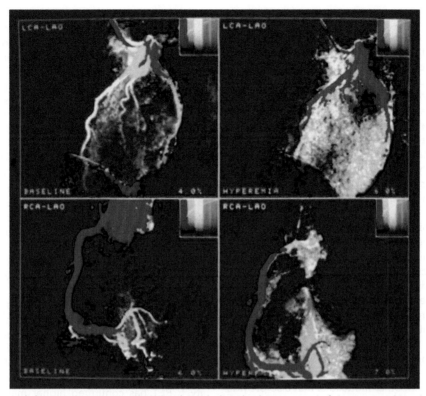

Fig. 2. Myocardial appearance time at angiography with digital enhancement. Left (*upper panels*) and right (*lower panels*) coronary systems are displayed at rest (*left panels*) and during hyperemia. (*From* Vogel R, LeFree M, Bates E, et al. Application of digital techniques to selective coronary arteriography: use of myocardial contrast appearance time to measure coronary flow reserve. Am Heart J 1984;107:153–64; with permission.)

contrast to reach a standardized distal coronary landmark in the culprit vessel, with length correction (CTFC) required for the left anterior descending artery (LAD).[7] A higher CTFC following thrombolysis is correlated with a higher CFR[8] as well as in-hospital and 30-day mortality.[9]

An attempt to angiographically visualize dye passing through the microcirculation can be made by establishing the degree of myocardial perfusion following angiographic injection with reasonable reproducibility and reliability. This is known as TIMI myocardial perfusion grading (TMPG). Following primary angioplasty, the degree of TPMG is correlated with mortality independent of the TFC.[10] Significantly, in patients with TIMI 3 flow following treatment of a myocardial infarction, an abnormal TPMG can be seen in up to two-thirds of patients and this has a significant impact on long-term mortality.[5,11] For example, in 924 subjects with TIMI 3 flow after a revascularized myocardial infarction a TPMG grade of 0 or 1 was associated with a higher mortality during the following 16 months.[12]

TMPG 0: Failure of dye to enter the microvasculature

TPMG 1: Dye enters slowly but fails to exit the microvasculature (still present at next injection)

TPMG 2: Delayed entry and exit from the microvasculature (persists after 3 cardiac cycles)

TPMG 3: Normal entry and exit from the microvasculature

However, although reasonably applicable, these direct-angiographic methods are relatively crude and subjective. Several studies have confirmed their insensitive nature. For example, a normal TFC can often be seen in patients with significant microvascular obstruction[13] or an abnormal CFR.[14] Therefore, more sophisticated techniques are required for an accurate assessment.

CORONARY FLOW RESERVE

CFR, the ratio of resting-to-hyperemic blood flow, was the one of earliest intravascular investigative tools implemented for assessing the coronary circulation. Of note, its first aim was to attempt to quantify coronary stenosis severity. Meticulous work by Gould and colleagues[15] demonstrated the effect of an increasing stenosis on resting and hyperemic flow rates. However, because of the variable influence of (particularly) the precapillary arterioles, it is difficult to use CFR to reliably assess coronary lesions. In contrast, controlling for epicardial resistance is relatively easy because in the absence of angiographically demonstrable disease the resistance of the large arteries of the heart is minimal and CFR provides information on the microvasculature alone.

Much discussion has gone into establishing the precise cut-off for an abnormal CFR, a value that has proved highly elusive. This is partly due to the continuous nature of the microcirculation in which, unlike coronary stenosis, no single value defines health versus disease. Additionally, almost all CFR-based studies have compared this value with other modalities that also provide a combined assessment of the macrovascular and microvascular circulation. Only a few, such as epicardial biopsy, focus on an alternative, microvascular-unique value.

Despite these issues, CFR as a tool for microcirculatory interrogation is one of the few intravascular investigative techniques that can be performed noninvasively through use of conventional echocardiography[16,17] (Fig. 3), myocardial contrast perfusion echocardiography,[18] or PET scanning.[19] This enhanced applicability allows for assessment of a much larger population than would be possible solely with invasive techniques and the conclusions that are drawn are also appropriate for any invasively obtained data.

CFR provides insights on the microcirculation in the postinfarct state. Following a revascularized myocardial infarction with TIMI 3 flow, a reduced CFR is associated with the presence of microvascular obstruction on MRI,[20] a feature in itself associated with a poorer prognosis[21] and infarct size.[22] Invasively measured CFR after primary percutaneous coronary intervention (PCI) therapy can predict the likelihood of ventricular recovery[23] and in-hospital mortality.[24]

In stable diabetic and prediabetic subjects, early microcirculatory abnormalities are recognizable as a low CFR.[25] An abnormal microcirculation has also been demonstrated with echocardiography-derived CFR in subjects with coronary syndrome X[16,26,27] and in subjects with multiple cardiovascular risk factors (hypertension, diabetes, obesity, impaired glucose tolerance) without overt coronary artery disease.[28] PET-derived CFR has been shown to be abnormal in hypertension,[29] diabetes,[30] hypercholesterolemia,[31] smoking,[32] left ventricular hypertrophy,[33] and aortic stenosis.[34]

Histologic comparisons have also been noted. There is a reasonable correlation between the presence of thin-cap fibroatheroma (on virtual histology–intravascular ultrasound) and an abnormal CFR, which indicates an important link between the pathogenetic processes of both epicardial and microvascular disease.[35] CFR is abnormally low in patients with idiopathic dilated cardiomyopathy[36] and correlates well with myocardial capillary density in this subgroup.[37]

CFR in stable patients also conveys important prognostic information. One of the largest prospective CFR studies was undertaken using transthoracic echocardiography of more than 4000 subjects in whom an abnormal LAD-CFR was an independent predictor of 4-year mortality.[38] PET has confirmed higher major adverse cardiac event rates in individuals with a low CFR over 10 years.[39] Alternatively, CFR from myocardial contrast perfusion echocardiography has been shown to be an independent predictor of myocardial infarction risk or death in 1252 subjects.[40]

In patients with coexisting intermediate coronary disease, the presence of an abnormal CFR is a significant risk factor for a major adverse cardiac event at 10 years, more so than an abnormal FFR, demonstrating the importance of both microvascular assessment and its involvement in outcome.[41] Similarly, in the Women's Ischemia Syndrome Evaluation (WISE) study, subjects with nonobstructive coronary disease but an abnormal coronary vasomotor response had a higher likelihood of events during the following 2 years.[42]

CFR can also quantify the microcirculatory impact within cardiomyopathic processes. In 129 subjects with a dilated cardiomyopathy of unknown cause and normal coronary arteries, a poor echocardiography-derived CFR is seen in up to 64% of subjects and is a predictor of adverse events (defined as worsening of heart failure symptoms or death).[43] An abnormal CFR is also a marker of poor outcome in hypertrophic cardiomyopathy (defined as left atrium dilatation, development of atrial fibrillation, hospitalization for unstable angina, implantable

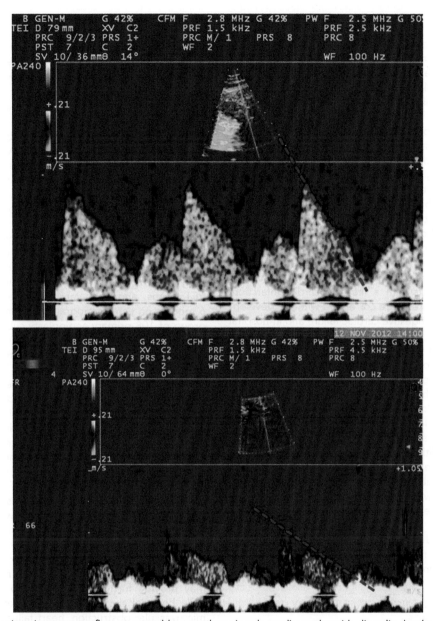

Fig. 3. Noninvasive coronary flow measured by transthoracic echocardiography with diastolic deceleration time marked in red. A more marked diastolic deceleration (*left panel*) is associated with poor microvascular function compared with the right panel. Alternatively or additionally, peripheral administration of a stressor agent would provide noninvasive CFR.

cardioverter defibrillator insertion, or permanent pacemaker insertion).[44]

However, despite the availability of CFR to interrogate the microcirculation, several caveats exist for its use. An increasing heart rate results in an higher resting coronary flow rate[45] but hyperemic rates are unchanged,[46,47] producing a relative reduction in CFR. Similarly, with volume expansion and a rise in pulmonary capillary wedge pressure, resting coronary flow rate is increased but hyperemic flow is unchanged,

again resulting in a reduction in CFR.[47] There is also physiologic variability with a higher resting coronary flow rate seen in women[48] and with age.[49] Various pharmacologic agents also exert an effect on CFR independent of heart rate alterations.[50] Therefore, whereas pressure-derived indices strive for an accurate definition of peak hyperemia,[51] with flow-based measures it is the definition of rest that creates more difficulties undoubtedly contributing to the precision issues of CFR.[52]

RESTING CORONARY FLOW PATTERNS

Interest has also focused on resting coronary flow patterns as a marker of myocardial dysfunction. Initial work examined the Doppler flow profile in 42 subjects after angioplasty for acute myocardial infarction and the presence of no-reflow on myocardial contrast echocardiography. Although peak diastolic velocity was the same in subjects with and without no-reflow, diastolic deceleration (see Fig. 3) was significantly higher in the latter. Additionally, early systolic retrograde coronary flow was noted in these subjects.[53] This feature is thought to reflect capillary damage (rather than microembolization).[54]

Diastolic deceleration time and early systolic flow reversal also correlate with TIMI flow[55] and their presence confers prognostic information. In 169 subjects with a first myocardial infarction, these features were correlated with the development of congestive cardiac failure and in-hospital mortality.[56] Using noninvasive Doppler in 49 subjects with a successfully reperfused artery, the presence of systolic flow reversal was associated with a poor recovery of left ventricular function on transthoracic echocardiography.[57] Invasive Doppler flow profiles 4 days after acute myocardial infarction were also able to predict the degree of microvascular obstruction seen on MRI.[58] Moreover, additional use of intracoronary streptokinase at the time of primary angioplasty seems to result in a favorable improvement in diastolic deceleration time when measured invasively 2 days later.[59] In a prospective 4-year follow-up of 68 myocardial infarction subjects, these flow patterns were associated with outcome in terms of cardiac death, recurrent myocardial infarction, and congestive heart failure.[60]

INDEX OF MICROCIRCULATORY RESISTANCE

Through use of sensor-tipped wires, thermodilution has been shown to be a useful tool for estimating CFR[61] and has been validated as such in humans.[62] By including a combined distal pressure measurement with hyperemic thermodilution-derived transit time, the index of microcirculatory resistance (IMR) is calculated as the product of both (Fig. 4). This has been validated in animals[63] and humans[64] as a reliable measure of microvascular function independent of hemodynamic perturbations.

IMR has been used in stable and unstable settings to provide valuable prognostic and diagnostic information. In patients undergoing elective angioplasty, IMR was able to predict the likelihood of periprocedural myocardial infarction[65] and show, therefore, that the status of the microcirculation is involved in this risk. IMR has also been used to demonstrate the advantages of direct stenting, which resulted in a lower IMR than if lesion pretreatment with balloon dilatation was used[66] (a feature also demonstrated with CTFC[67]). Intracoronary angiotensin-converting enzyme (ACE)-inhibitors[68] or pretreatment with atorvastatin[69] for elective PCI also result in a more favorable post-angioplasty IMR, implying that these adjuvant therapies offer microcirculatory protection to any iatrogenic showers of atheroma.

IMR has an important role in unstable patients. In a study of 40 subjects who underwent primary angioplasty, IMR performed immediately afterward correlated well with viability on PET scans and left ventricular recovery at 6 months on echocardiography.[70] Similarly, in a group of 108 primary angioplasty subjects, IMR was correlated with early (2 days) and late (3 months) myocardial salvage at MRI (defined as the ratio of infarct to area at risk).[71] A second study of 57 STEMI subjects also showed a significant correlation between MRI-derived microvascular obstruction and periprocedural IMR.[72] IMR has been used to demonstrate the time course of microvascular recovery after myocardial infarction with a gradual improvement noted during the following 6 months in hyperemic transit time, CFR, and IMR.[20]

In the largest study of infarct-measured IMR, Fearon and colleagues[73] have shown that in 253 subjects an IMR of greater than 40 is an independent predictor of death or rehospitalization for heart failure during a 2.8 year follow-up. Finally, the shape of the thermodilution curve may provide further prognostic information; a wide bimodal shape predicts the likelihood of microvascular obstruction, heart failure rehospitalization, or death.[74]

IMR has a use in guiding adjuvant therapies at the time of primary angioplasty. Nicorandil, a nitric oxide donor, has a positive effect during myocardial infarction in which a consecutive reduction in microvascular resistance was seen with repeat administrations of intracoronary nicorandil. IMR also correlated well with TFC, myocardial blush grade, and peak creatine kinase.[75] Future research is planned to examine the effect of antiplatelet agents on microvascular function (as assessed by IMR) in acute coronary syndrome.[76]

In a study of 41 subjects randomized to receive intracoronary streptokinase at primary PCI, IMR was repeated after 2 days. Subjects in

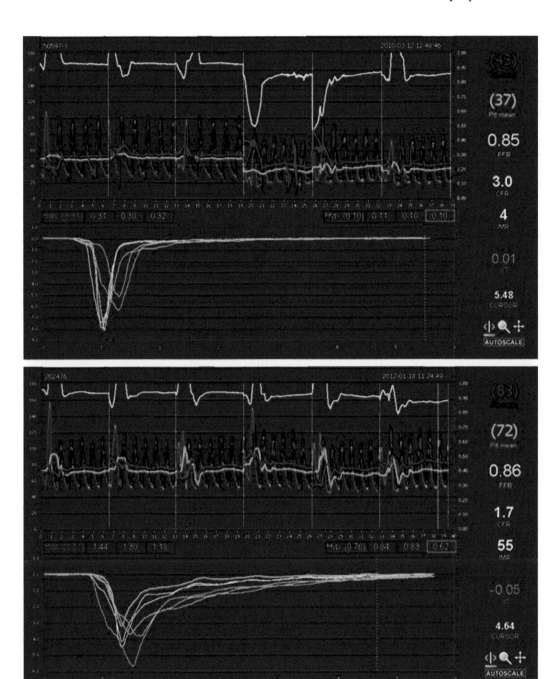

Fig. 4. The index of microvascular resistance in health and disease. The upper panel demonstrates a healthy vasculature with a low index of microcirculatory resistance (IMR) and high CFR. The lower panel demonstrates an unhealthy microvasculature with a high IMR and low CFR.

the streptokinase arm had significantly lower IMR levels (16 vs 32) although no differences were seen between these groups on echocardiography or PET scan.[59] A similar study of 36 STEMI subjects randomized to receive or not receive distal protection during angioplasty

showed similar results; those who received distal protection the IMR also had significantly lower IMR levels (27 vs 37).[77]

The potential usefulness of IMR compared with CFR has been demonstrated in a study of 25 heart transplant subjects. Although CFR was unchanged when measured after transplantation and at 1 year, FFR significantly worsened whereas IMR significantly improved. This implies that unfavorable epicardial changes occurred in conjunction with more favorable and opposing microcirculatory alterations. Because CFR is related to both epicardial and microvascular disease, if divergent changes occur, it is not able to distinguish these. Therefore, techniques that independently assess the microvasculature are much more informative in this setting.[78]

INSTANTANEOUS HYPEREMIC DIASTOLIC VELOCITY-PRESSURE SLOPE

Due to the inherent problems with CFR outlined previously, Mancini and colleagues[79] examined the relationship between pressure and flow during diastole under hyperemic conditions, measuring the pressure-volume slope during mid-diastole to late-diastole (Fig. 5) as a tool for stenosis assessment. In animal models, the instantaneous hyperemic diastolic velocity-pressure slope (IHDVPS) proved to be independent of hemodynamic variables, well-correlated with microsphere-derived coronary conductance (the inverse of resistance),[80] reproducible, and potentially more sensitive than CFR to epicardial stenosis.[81] It was also insensitive to changes in heart rate, contractility, and volume loading.[82]

Di Mario and colleagues[83] moved IHDVPS into the clinical environment in a study of 95 subjects, albeit still for epicardial stenosis severity assessment. Again, little effect was exerted by alteration in hemodynamic conditions and a reasonable correlation was obtained with stenosis severity, which was echoed by findings 2 years later.[84]

Subsequently, this technique was applied to assessing the microcirculation. Using a cohort of subjects who had undergone previous cardiac

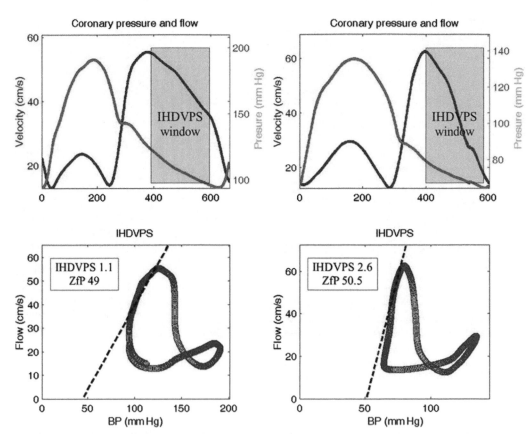

Fig. 5. Calculation of the coronary zero flow pressure and instantaneous hyperemic diastolic velocity-pressure slope (IHDVPS) in 2 patients (*right* and *left panels*). The slope of the diastolic relationship between pressure and flow provides a measure of conductance (the inverse of resistance). The x-intercept is the zero-flow pressure (ZFP). Both patients have a markedly elevated similar ZFP; however, the right panel displays a more favorable IHDVPS and thus lower resistance than the left panel. In the context of a myocardial infarction, both are likely to have an elevated left ventricular end-diastolic pressure; BP, blood pressure.

transplantation, Escaned and colleagues[85] performed simultaneous myocardial biopsy and intracoronary interrogation, thus linking physiologic indices with histologic findings. Notably, a good correlation was demonstrated with capillary density and arteriolar obliteration, although no link was demonstrated between histology and CFR. The same group also demonstrated a link between diastolic dysfunction in diabetic subjects and IHDVPS but not zero-flow pressure (ZFP).[86] Therefore, in the absence of coronary stenosis, IHDVPS seems to be a good tool for detecting microcirculatory changes.

The coronary pressure-volume loop also seems to be useful in acute myocardial infarction. In 27 subjects with anterior myocardial infarctions, both IHDVPS and ZFP correlated with myocardial viability on fluorodeoxyglucose (FDG)-PET scan (although IHDVPS did not quite reach significance).[87] Peri-infarct IHDVPS also correlates with the degree of myocardial salvage on technetium sestamibi (MIBI) scan,[88] the transmural extent of infarction on MRI,[89] and the likelihood of left ventricular remodeling.[90]

An elucidating study published by Van Herck and colleagues[91] used the model of myocardial infarction to demonstrate the dominant influence on ZFP. By comparing subjects with angina, non-Q wave infarction, and Q-wave infarction, a step-wise right-shift in the coronary flow relationship was demonstrated, a feature present in noninfarcted territory as well. Multivariate analysis showed that left ventricular end-diastolic pressure (LVEDP) was the most important determinant of ZFP. One caveat with the pressure-flow loop–derived ZFP was recognized by Di Mario and colleagues,[83] who suggested the relationship may become curvilinear at lower pressures, potentially hampering its use.

WAVE INTENSITY ANALYSIS

Initially developed as a tool in sound engineering and fluid dynamics, wave intensity analysis (WIA) has found a particular place in assessing the coronary microcirculation. It is derived from simultaneously acquired resting measures of pressure and flow. Unlike traditional Fourier-based interrogation of waveform data, it is calculated in the time-domain.[92] At its most basic level, net wave intensity (WI_{NET}) is constructed from the product of the first differential of pressure and flow:

$$WI_{NET} = dP \times dU$$

However, by incorporating the water-hammer equations and by standardizing by time it is able to provide the direction of origin of the separated force:

$$WI_{\pm} = 1/4\rho c \times (dP/dt \pm \rho c dU/dt)$$

ρc, where ρ is the density of blood and c is wave speed (itself calculated from a single measure of pressure and flow[93]). Coronary wave intensity is, therefore, able to separate out the proximal (aortic) and distal (myocardial) originating energy components that contribute to accelerate and decelerate coronary flow and provides an independent measure of the energy being exerted from the myocardium.

Although 6 waves have been identified per cardiac cycle, the dominant wave affecting coronary flow is the backward decompression wave (**Fig. 6**).[94] This wave was initially referred to as a suction wave, which reflects its mechanistic contribution because, as the microcirculation relaxes in diastole, a negative pressure gradient is created from the recoiling capillaries sucking blood into the microcirculation.

The microcirculation has been examined in various states using WIA. First, in left ventricular hypertrophy, a negative effect is seen on the backward decompression wave, reflecting the relative inefficiency of this state.[94] In severe aortic stenosis, despite the presence of significant left ventricular hypertrophy, the backward decompression wave is greatly increased due to the increased compression and relaxation necessary to expel blood through the stenotic aortic valve.[95] With pacing in severe aortic stenosis, the backward decompression wave decreases with an increased heart rate, reflecting a relative uncoupling of the normal mechanisms governing coronary blood flow and possibly accounting for angina in these patients. Importantly, this relationship returns to the physiologic norm immediately after transcatheter valve implantation.[95]

WIA has also been used in patients with coronary artery disease to investigate the phenomenon of warm-up angina in which an improvement in the cardiac-coronary coupling is seen with consecutive exertions.[96] The same group also used WIA to predict the likelihood of myocardial recovery on MRI after 3 months in 31 subjects who underwent revascularization following a non-STEMI.[97]

In biventricularly paced patients, optimization of the pacing regime (as determined by noninvasive blood pressure measurements) resulted in an increase in coronary blood flow velocity due to an increase in the backward decompression

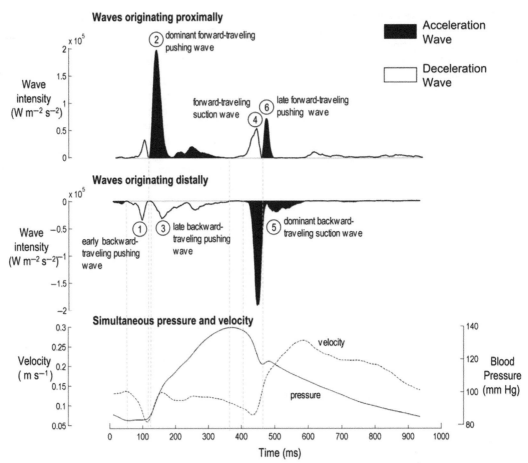

Fig. 6. Wave intensity profile in an unobstructed circumflex artery. Six waves are evident but the backward traveling suction or decompression wave (5) is responsible for coronary flow. This wave is generated by myocardial decompression at the onset of diastole. A pressure gradient is created from proximal to distal and this wave, therefore, provides a separated quantification of microvascular function. (*From* Davies JE, Whinnett ZI, Francis DP, et al. Evidence of a dominant backward-propagating "suction" wave responsible for diastolic coronary filling in humans, attenuated in left ventricular hypertrophy. Circulation 2006;113:1768–78; with permission.)

wave.[98] Finally, by documenting the wave-intensity profile of patients with moderate coronary lesions, a region of the cardiac cycle in which microvascular resistance is naturally low can be located and thus adenosine-free pressure-based assessment of coronary lesions can be performed.[99]

SUMMARY

The coronary microcirculation represents a vast network of conduits that cannot be directly visualized during angiography but whose role in channeling and regulating myocardial blood flow is paramount. Microcirculatory dysfunction is recognized in several clinical scenarios ranging from ischemia in the absence of epicardial stenosis, inherited cardiomyopathies, and acute myocardial infarction. Tools to investigate the microcirculation are not only essential for diagnostic purposes but also to guide treatment, particularly adjuvant therapies (such as thrombus aspiration or intracoronary pharmacotherapy) that may be required at the time of infarction. As such, the ability to assess the microcirculation using technology that can be applied at the time of angiography is essential to advancing the management of these conditions.

Although a basic understanding of the state of the microcirculation can be established from relatively direct angiographic markers, it is now obvious that, even in the presence of a normal blush grade or TIMI flow, significant abnormalities can still exist in the microcirculation. The resting coronary flow pattern is a more discriminatory tool and its use can predict outcome particularly by measuring the diastolic deceleration time and systolic flow reversal.

More sophisticated techniques rely on the induction of hyperemia to minimize microvascular tone. CFR measured in the absence of an epicardial stenosis allows direct assessment of the microcirculation. However, its variability with heart rate, volume status, age, and sex introduce several confounding factors. Despite this, CFR is one of the more widely applied and historically embedded techniques that can be replicated noninvasively. Therefore, it remains a potentially useful and applicable tool, particularly if ways of controlling for these confounding factors can be established.

To that end, IMR seems to be a promising thermodilution-based assessment technique involving simultaneous measures of pressure and thermodilution transit time with several documented advantages compared with CFR. However, it has some conceptual issues when coronary disease coexists owing to the presence of collateral flow. It requires either the measurement of coronary wedge pressure[100] or additional mathematical steps,[101] which add either complexity to the measurement or the potential to introduce error.

An alternate measure that combines hyperemic pressure and flow is IHDVPS, which has similar advantages compared with CFR due to its stability within varying hemodynamic states. However, achieving an optimal flow signal during hyperemia does require some skill and any pressure damping due to aggressive catheter engagement with the increased flow will have a marked effect. Additionally, there is concern about the use of the ZFP from the pressure-volume slope owing to the potential curvilinear relationship of pressure during low flow.[83]

WIA is able to assess the microcirculation in the resting state and incorporates measures of wave speed and blood density, as well as the pressure and flow waveforms. Although mathematically complex, when performed correctly it is able to provide independent information regarding microcirculatory function in the absence of a vasodilator. It has some disadvantages, particularly because, currently, no commercial software exists to provide a live measure and analysis is performed offline. Additionally, given its complex nature, there is a danger for error-exaggeration and some questions exist about how the data should be mathematically processed.[102] There is also some debate about the single-point equation for establishing wave speed, which, certainly during hyperemia, may not be as sound.[103]

In summary, as these techniques are applied and developed it is apparent that a single technique is unlikely to provide a complete comprehensive assessment of the microcirculation. Therefore, the future of intravascular assessment of the coronary microcirculation will most likely involve several complementary modalities ideally deployed simultaneously. As such, both wave-intensity analysis and IHDVPS can be gathered from a single pressure- and flow-tipped wire during periods of hyperemia and rest along with the more conventional measure of CFR. These may, therefore, integrate easily and synergistically. However, in the presence of significant epicardial disease, IMR also allows calculation of the FFR and this dual assessment tool may be more appropriate in this setting.

REFERENCES

1. Chilian WM, Eastham CL, Marcus ML. Microvascular distribution of coronary vascular resistance in beating left ventricle. Am J Physiol 1986;251: H779–88.
2. Nellis SH, Liedtke AJ, Whitesell L. Small coronary vessel pressure and diameter in an intact beating rabbit heart using fixed-position and free-motion techniques. Circ Res 1981;49:342–53.
3. Vogel R, LeFree M, Bates E, et al. Application of digital techniques to selective coronary arteriography: use of myocardial contrast appearance time to measure coronary flow reserve. Am Heart J 1984;107:153–64.
4. Kern MJ, Moore JA, Aguirre FV, et al. Determination of angiographic (TIMI grade) blood flow by intracoronary Doppler flow velocity during acute myocardial infarction. Circulation 1996;94: 1545–52.
5. Gibson CM, Cannon CP, Murphy SA, et al. Relationship of TIMI myocardial perfusion grade to mortality after administration of thrombolytic drugs. Circulation 2000;101:125–30.
6. Anderson JL, Karagounis LA, Califf RM. Metaanalysis of five reported studies on the relation of early coronary patency grades with mortality and outcomes after acute myocardial infarction. Am J Cardiol 1996;78:1–8.
7. Gibson CM, Cannon CP, Daley WL, et al. TIMI frame count: a quantitative method of assessing coronary artery flow. Circulation 1996;93:879–88.
8. Ishihara M, Sato H, Tateishi H, et al. Impaired coronary flow reserve immediately after coronary angioplasty in patients with acute myocardial infarction. Br Heart J 1993;69:288–92.
9. Gibson CM, Murphy SA, Rizzo MJ, et al. Relationship between TIMI frame count and clinical outcomes after thrombolytic administration. Circulation 1999;99:1945–50.

10. van 't Hof AWJ, Liem A, Suryapranata H, et al. Angiographic assessment of myocardial reperfusion in patients treated with primary angioplasty for acute myocardial infarction: myocardial blush grade. Circulation 1998;97:2302–6.

11. Stone GW, Peterson MA, Lansky AJ, et al. Impact of normalized myocardial perfusion after successful angioplasty in acute myocardial infarction. J Am Coll Cardiol 2002;39:591–7.

12. Henriques JPS, Zijlstra F, van 't Hof AWJ, et al. Angiographic assessment of reperfusion in acute myocardial infarction by myocardial blush grade. Circulation 2003;107:2115–9.

13. Nijveldt R, Beek AM, Hirsch A, et al. Functional recovery after acute myocardial infarction: comparison between angiography, electrocardiography, and cardiovascular magnetic resonance measures of microvascular injury. J Am Coll Cardiol 2008;52:181–9.

14. Ohara Y, Hiasa Y, Takahashi T, et al. Relation between the TIMI frame count and the degree of microvascular injury after primary coronary angioplasty in patients with acute anterior myocardial infarction. Heart 2005;91:64–7.

15. Gould KL, Lipscomb K, Hamilton GW. Physiologic basis for assessing critical coronary stenosis: instantaneous flow response and regional distribution during coronary hyperemia as measures of coronary flow reserve. Am J Cardiol 1974;33:87–94.

16. Rigo F. Coronary flow reserve in stress-echo lab. From pathophysiologic toy to diagnostic tool. Cardiovasc Ultrasound 2005;3:8.

17. Rigo F, Tona FR, Cati A, et al. Coronary flow velocity assessment on left anterior coronary artery as a marker of atherosclerosis: reliability and accuracy of transthoracic echocardiographic study compared to Doppler flow wire. Eur Heart J 2010;31:254.

18. Wei K, Ragosta M, Thorpe J, et al. Noninvasive quantification of coronary blood flow reserve in humans using myocardial contrast echocardiography. Circulation 2001;103:2560–5.

19. Schindler TH, Zhang X-L, Mhiri L, et al. Role of PET in the evaluation and understanding of coronary physiology. J Nucl Cardiol 2007;14:589–603.

20. Cuculi F, De Maria GL, Meier P, et al. Impact of microvascular obstruction on the assessment of coronary flow reserve, index of microcirculatory resistance, and fractional flow reserve after ST-segment elevation myocardial infarction. J Am Coll Cardiol 2014;64:1894–904.

21. Klug G, Mayr A, Schenk S, et al. Prognostic value at 5 years of microvascular obstruction after acute myocardial infarction assessed by cardiovascular magnetic resonance. J Cardiovasc Magn Reson 2012;14:46.

22. de Waard G, Teunissen PF, Hollander MR, et al. Abstract 20337: implications of invasively measured coronary flow reserve on infarct size directly following reperfusion after acute myocardial infarction in both humans and an experimental pig model. Circulation 2014;130:A20337.

23. Lepper W, Hoffmann R, Kamp O, et al. Assessment of myocardial reperfusion by intravenous myocardial contrast echocardiography and coronary flow reserve after primary percutaneous transluminal coronary angioplasty [correction of angiography] in patients with acute myocardial infarction. Circulation 2000;101:2368–74.

24. Meimoun P, Malaquin D, Benali T, et al. Non-invasive coronary flow reserve after successful primary angioplasty for acute anterior myocardial infarction is an independent predictor of left ventricular recovery and in-hospital cardiac events. J Am Soc Echocardiogr 2009;22:1071–9.

25. Erdogan D, Yucel H, Uysal BA, et al. Effects of pre-diabetes and diabetes on left ventricular and coronary microvascular functions. Metabolism 2013; 62:1123–30.

26. Zehetgruber M, Mundigler G, Christ G, et al. Estimation of coronary flow reserve by transesophageal coronary sinus Doppler measurements in patients with syndrome X and patients with significant left coronary artery disease. J Am Coll Cardiol 1995; 25:1039–45.

27. Galiuto L, Sestito A, Barchetta S, et al. Non-invasive evaluation of flow reserve in the left anterior descending coronary artery in patients with cardiac syndrome X. Am J Cardiol 2007;99: 1378–83.

28. Pirat B, Bozbas H, Simsek V, et al. Impaired coronary flow reserve in patients with metabolic syndrome. Atherosclerosis 2008;201:112–6.

29. Neglia D, Fommei E, Varela-Carver A, et al. Perindopril and indapamide reverse coronary microvascular remodelling and improve flow in arterial hypertension. J Hypertens 2011;29:364–72.

30. Prior JO, Quinones MJ, Hernandez-Pampaloni M, et al. Coronary circulatory dysfunction in insulin resistance, impaired glucose tolerance, and type 2 diabetes mellitus. Circulation 2005;111:2291–8.

31. Yokoyama I, Ohtake T, Momomura S, et al. Reduced coronary flow reserve in hypercholesterolemic patients without overt coronary stenosis. Circulation 1996;94:3232–8.

32. Kaufmann PA, Gnecchi-Ruscone T, di Terlizzi M, et al. Coronary heart disease in smokers: vitamin C restores coronary microcirculatory function. Circulation 2000;102:1233–8.

33. Choudhury L, Rosen SD, Patel D, et al. Coronary vasodilator reserve in primary and secondary left ventricular hypertrophy. A study with positron emission tomography. Eur Heart J 1997;18:108–16.

34. Rajappan K, Rimoldi OE, Camici PG, et al. Functional changes in coronary microcirculation after

valve replacement in patients with aortic stenosis. Circulation 2003;107:3170–5.

35. Dhawan SS, Corban MT, Nanjundappa RA, et al. Coronary microvascular dysfunction is associated with higher frequency of thin-cap fibroatheroma. Atherosclerosis 2012;223:384–8.

36. Canetti M, Akhter MW, Lerman A, et al. Evaluation of myocardial blood flow reserve in patients with chronic congestive heart failure due to idiopathic dilated cardiomyopathy. Am J Cardiol 2003;92:1246–9.

37. Tsagalou EP, Anastasiou-Nana M, Agapitos E, et al. Depressed coronary flow reserve is associated with decreased myocardial capillary density in patients with heart failure due to idiopathic dilated cardiomyopathy. J Am Coll Cardiol 2008;52:1391–8.

38. Cortigiani L, Rigo F, Gherardi S, et al. Coronary flow reserve during dipyridamole stress echocardiography predicts mortality. JACC Cardiovasc Imaging 2012;5:1079–85.

39. Herzog BA, Husmann L, Valenta I, et al. Long-term prognostic value of 13N-ammonia myocardial perfusion positron emission tomography added value of coronary flow reserve. J Am Coll Cardiol 2009;54:150–6.

40. Gaibazzi N, Reverberi C, Lorenzoni V, et al. Prognostic value of high-dose dipyridamole stress myocardial contrast perfusion echocardiography. Circulation 2012;126:1217–24.

41. van de Hoef TP, van Lavieren MA, Damman P, et al. Physiological basis and long-term clinical outcome of discordance between fractional flow reserve and coronary flow velocity reserve in coronary stenoses of intermediate severity. Circ Cardiovasc Interv 2014;7:301–11.

42. von Mering GO, Arant CB, Wessel TR, et al. Abnormal coronary vasomotion as a prognostic indicator of cardiovascular events in women: results from the National Heart, Lung, and Blood Institute-Sponsored Women's Ischemia Syndrome Evaluation (WISE). Circulation 2004;109:722–5.

43. Rigo F, Gherardi S, Galderisi M, et al. The prognostic impact of coronary flow-reserve assessed by Doppler echocardiography in non-ischaemic dilated cardiomyopathy. Eur Heart J 2006;27:1319–23.

44. Rigo F, Cortigiani L, Gherardi S, et al. Coronary microvascular dysfunction and prognosis in hypertrophic cardiomyopathy: a Doppler echocardiography study. Circulation 2007;116:369.

45. Duncker DJ, Bache RJ. Regulation of coronary blood flow during exercise. Physiol Rev 2008;88:1009–86.

46. Rossen JD, Winniford MD. Effect of increases in heart rate and arterial pressure on coronary flow reserve in humans. J Am Coll Cardiol 1993;21:343–8.

47. McGinn AL, White CW, Wilson RF. Interstudy variability of coronary flow reserve. Influence of heart rate, arterial pressure, and ventricular preload. Circulation 1990;81:1319–30.

48. Chareonthaitawee P, Kaufmann PA, Rimoldi O, et al. Heterogeneity of resting and hyperemic myocardial blood flow in healthy humans. Cardiovasc Res 2001;50:151–61.

49. Galderisi M, Rigo F, Gherardi S, et al. The impact of aging and atherosclerotic risk factors on transthoracic coronary flow reserve in subjects with normal coronary angiography. Cardiovasc Ultrasound 2012;10:20.

50. Skalidis EI, Hamilos MI, Chlouverakis G, et al. Ivabradine improves coronary flow reserve in patients with stable coronary artery disease. Atherosclerosis 2011;215:160–5.

51. Tarkin JM, Nijjer S, Sen S, et al. Hemodynamic response to intravenous adenosine and its effect on fractional flow reserve assessment: results of the Adenosine for the Functional Evaluation of Coronary Stenosis Severity (AFFECTS) study. Circ Cardiovasc Interv 2013;6(6):654–61.

52. Fearon WF. Assessing intermediate coronary lesions: more than meets the eye. Circulation 2013;128:2551–3.

53. Iwakura K, Ito H, Takiuchi S, et al. Alternation in the coronary blood flow velocity pattern in patients with no reflow and reperfused acute myocardial infarction. Circulation 1996;94:1269–75.

54. Yamamoto K, Ito H, Iwakura K, et al. Two different coronary blood flow velocity patterns in thrombolysis in myocardial infarction flow grade 2 in acute myocardial infarction: insight into mechanisms of microvascular dysfunction. J Am Coll Cardiol 2002;40:1755–60.

55. Akasaka T, Yoshida K, Kawamoto T, et al. Relation of phasic coronary flow velocity characteristics with TIMI perfusion grade and myocardial recovery after primary percutaneous transluminal coronary angioplasty and rescue stenting. Circulation 2000;101:2361–7.

56. Yamamuro A, Akasaka T, Tamita K, et al. Coronary flow velocity pattern immediately after percutaneous coronary intervention as a predictor of complications and in-hospital survival after acute myocardial infarction. Circulation 2002;106:3051–6.

57. Nohtomi Y, Takeuchi M, Nagasawa K, et al. Persistence of systolic coronary flow reversal predicts irreversible dysfunction after reperfused anterior myocardial infarction. Heart 2003;89:382–8.

58. Hirsch A, Nijveldt R, Haeck JD, et al. Relation between the assessment of microvascular injury by cardiovascular magnetic resonance and coronary Doppler flow velocity measurements in patients with acute anterior wall myocardial infarction. J Am Coll Cardiol 2008;51:2230–8.

59. Sezer M, Oflaz H, Gören T, et al. Intracoronary streptokinase after primary percutaneous coronary intervention. N Engl J Med 2007;356:1823–34.

60. Furber AP, Prunier F, Nguyen HCP, et al. Coronary blood flow assessment after successful angioplasty for acute myocardial infarction predicts the risk of long-term cardiac events. Circulation 2004;110:3527–33.

61. De Bruyne B, Pijls NH, Smith L, et al. Coronary thermodilution to assess flow reserve: experimental validation. Circulation 2001;104:2003–6.

62. Pijls NH, De Bruyne B, Smith L, et al. Coronary thermodilution to assess flow reserve: validation in humans. Circulation 2002;105:2482–6.

63. Fearon WF, Balsam LB, Farouque HMO, et al. Novel index for invasively assessing the coronary microcirculation. Circulation 2003;107:3129–32.

64. Ng MK, Yeung AC, Fearon WF. Invasive assessment of the coronary microcirculation: superior reproducibility and less hemodynamic dependence of index of microcirculatory resistance compared with coronary flow reserve. Circulation 2006;113:2054–61.

65. Ng MKC, Yong ASC, Ho M, et al. The index of microcirculatory resistance predicts myocardial infarction related to percutaneous coronary intervention. Circ Cardiovasc Interv 2012;5:515–22.

66. Cuisset T, Hamilos M, Melikian N, et al. Direct stenting for stable angina pectoris is associated with reduced periprocedural microcirculatory injury compared with stenting after pre-dilation. J Am Coll Cardiol 2008;51:1060–5.

67. Ozdemir R, Sezgin AT, Barutcu I, et al. Comparison of direct stenting versus conventional stent implantation on blood flow in patients with ST-segment elevation myocardial infarction. Angiology 2006;57:453–8.

68. Mangiacapra F, Peace AJ, Di Serafino L, et al. Intracoronary EnalaPrilat to Reduce MICROvascular Damage During Percutaneous Coronary Intervention (ProMicro) study. J Am Coll Cardiol 2013;61:615–21.

69. Fujii K, Kawasaki D, Oka K, et al. The impact of pravastatin pre-treatment on periprocedural microcirculatory damage in patients undergoing percutaneous coronary intervention. JACC Cardiovasc Interv 2011;4:513–20.

70. Lim H-S, Yoon M-H, Tahk S-J, et al. Usefulness of the index of microcirculatory resistance for invasively assessing myocardial viability immediately after primary angioplasty for anterior myocardial infarction. Eur Heart J 2009;30:2854–60.

71. Payne AR, Berry C, Doolin O, et al. Microvascular resistance predicts myocardial salvage and infarct characteristics in ST-elevation myocardial infarction. J Am Heart Assoc 2012;1:e002246.

72. McGeoch R, Watkins S, Berry C, et al. The index of microcirculatory resistance measured acutely predicts the extent and severity of myocardial infarction in patients with ST-segment elevation myocardial infarction. JACC Cardiovasc Interv 2010;3:715–22.

73. Fearon WF, Low AF, Yong AS, et al. Prognostic value of the index of microcirculatory resistance measured after primary percutaneous coronary intervention. Circulation 2013;127:2436–41.

74. Fukunaga M, Fujii K, Kawasaki D, et al. Thermodilution-derived coronary blood flow pattern immediately after coronary intervention as a predictor of microcirculatory damage and midterm clinical outcomes in patients with ST-segment-elevation myocardial infarction. Circ Cardiovasc Interv 2014;7:149–55.

75. Ito N, Nanto S, Doi Y, et al. Beneficial effects of intracoronary nicorandil on microvascular dysfunction after primary percutaneous coronary intervention: demonstration of its superiority to nitroglycerin in a cross-over study. Cardiovasc Drugs Ther 2013;27:279–87.

76. Park SD, Baek YS, Woo SI, et al. Comparing the effect of clopidogrel versus ticagrelor on coronary microvascular dysfunction in acute coronary syndrome patients (TIME trial): study protocol for a randomized controlled trial. Trials 2014;15:151.

77. Ito N, Nanto S, Doi Y, et al. Distal protection during primary coronary intervention can preserve the index of microcirculatory resistance in patients with acute anterior ST-segment elevation myocardial infarction. Circ J 2011;75:94–8.

78. Fearon WF, Hirohata A, Nakamura M, et al. Discordant changes in epicardial and microvascular coronary physiology after cardiac transplantation: Physiologic Investigation for Transplant Arteriopathy II (PITA II) study. J Heart Lung Transplant 2006;25:765–71.

79. Mancini GB, McGillem MJ, DeBoe SF, et al. The diastolic hyperemic flow versus pressure relation. A new index of coronary stenosis severity and flow reserve. Circulation 1989;80:941–50.

80. Mancini GB, Cleary RM, DeBoe SF, et al. Instantaneous hyperemic flow-versus-pressure slope index. Microsphere validation of an alternative to measures of coronary reserve. Circulation 1991; 84:862–70.

81. Cleary RM, Moore NB, DeBoe SF, et al. Sensitivity and reproducibility of the instantaneous hyperemic flow versus pressure slope index compared to coronary flow reserve for the assessment of stenosis severity. Am Heart J 1993;126:57–65.

82. Cleary RM, Ayon D, Moore NB, et al. Tachycardia, contractility and volume loading alter conventional indexes of coronary flow reserve, but not the instantaneous hyperemic flow versus pressure slope index. J Am Coll Cardiol 1992;20: 1261–9.

83. Di Mario C, Krams R, Gil R, et al. Slope of the instantaneous hyperemic diastolic coronary flow velocity-pressure relation. A new index for assessment of the physiological significance of coronary stenosis in humans. Circulation 1994;90:1215–24.

84. Kondo M, Azuma A, Yamada H, et al. Estimation of coronary flow reserve with the instantaneous coronary flow velocity versus pressure relation: a new index of coronary flow reserve independent of perfusion pressure. Am Heart J 1996;132:1127–34.

85. Escaned J, Flores A, Garcia-Pavia P, et al. Assessment of microcirculatory remodeling with intracoronary flow velocity and pressure measurements: validation with endomyocardial sampling in cardiac allografts. Circulation 2009;120:1561–8.

86. Escaned J, Colmenarez H, Ferrer MC, et al. Diastolic dysfunction in diabetic patients assessed with Doppler echocardiography: relationship with coronary atherosclerotic burden and microcirculatory impairment. Rev Esp Cardiol 2009;62:1395–403.

87. Shimada K, Sakanoue Y, Kobayashi Y, et al. Assessment of myocardial viability using coronary zero flow pressure after successful angioplasty in patients with acute anterior myocardial infarction. Heart 2003;89:71–6.

88. Shibata T, Watanabe H, Tsurusaki T, et al. Do indices of coronary conductance after reperfusion reflect the extent of salvaged myocardium? Jpn Heart J 2004;45:387–96.

89. Kitabata H, Imanishi T, Kubo T, et al. Coronary microvascular resistance index immediately after primary percutaneous coronary intervention as a predictor of the transmural extent of infarction in patients with ST-segment elevation anterior acute myocardial infarction. JACC Cardiovasc Imaging 2009;2:263–72.

90. Kitabata H, Kubo T, Ishibashi K, et al. Prognostic value of microvascular resistance index immediately after primary percutaneous coronary intervention on left ventricular remodeling in patients with reperfused anterior acute ST-segment elevation myocardial infarction. JACC Cardiovasc Interventions 2013;6:1046–54.

91. Van Herck PL, Carlier SG, Claeys MJ, et al. Coronary microvascular dysfunction after myocardial infarction: increased coronary zero flow pressure both in the infarcted and in the remote myocardium is mainly related to left ventricular filling pressure. Heart 2007;93:1231–7.

92. Parker KH. An introduction to wave intensity analysis. Med Biol Eng Comput 2009;47:175–88.

93. Davies JE, Whinnett ZI, Francis DP, et al. Use of simultaneous pressure and velocity measurements to estimate arterial wave speed at a single site in humans. Am J Physiol Heart Circ Physiol 2006;290:H878–85.

94. Davies JE, Whinnett ZI, Francis DP, et al. Evidence of a dominant backward-propagating "suction" wave responsible for diastolic coronary filling in humans, attenuated in left ventricular hypertrophy. Circulation 2006;113:1768–78.

95. Davies JE, Sen S, Broyd C, et al. Arterial pulse wave dynamics after percutaneous aortic valve replacement/clinical perspective. Circulation 2011;124:1565–72.

96. Lockie TP, Rolandi MC, Guilcher A, et al. Synergistic adaptations to exercise in the systemic and coronary circulations that underlie the warm-up angina phenomenon. Circulation 2012;126:2565–74.

97. Silva KD, Guilcher A, Lockie T, et al. Coronary wave intensity: a novel invasive tool for predicting myocardial viability following acute coronary syndromes. J Am Coll Cardiol 2012;59:E421–2.

98. Kyriacou A, Whinnett ZI, Sen S, et al. Improvement in coronary blood flow velocity with acute biventricular pacing is predominantly due to an increase in a diastolic backward-travelling decompression (suction) wave. Circulation 2012;126:1334–44.

99. Sen S, Escaned J, Malik IS, et al. Development and validation of a new adenosine-independent index of stenosis severity from coronary wave–intensity analysis: results of the ADVISE (ADenosine Vasodilator Independent Stenosis Evaluation) Study. J Am Coll Cardiol 2012;59:1392–402.

100. Layland J, MacIsaac AI, Burns AT, et al. When collateral supply is accounted for epicardial stenosis does not increase microvascular resistance. Circ Cardiovasc Interv 2012;5:97–102.

101. Yong AS, Layland J, Fearon WF, et al. Calculation of the index of microcirculatory resistance without coronary wedge pressure measurement in the presence of epicardial stenosis. JACC Cardiovasc Interventions 2013;6:53–8.

102. Rivolo S, Nagel E, Smith NP, et al. Automatic selection of optimal Savitzky-Golay filter parameters for Coronary Wave Intensity Analysis. Conf Proc IEEE Eng Med Biol Soc 2014;2014:5056–9.

103. Rolandi MC, De Silva K, Lumley M, et al. Wave speed in human coronary arteries is not influenced by microvascular vasodilation: implications for wave intensity analysis. Basic Res Cardiol 2014;109:405.

Can Resting Indices Obviate the Need for Hyperemia and Promote the Routine Use of Physiologically Guided Revascularization?

Sayan Sen, BSc, MBBS, MRCP, PhD*, Ricardo Petraco, MD, MRCP,
Sukhjinder Nijjer, BSc, MBChB, MRCP, Jamil Mayet, MD, FESC,
Justin Davies, BSc, MBBS, MRCP, PhD

KEYWORDS

• iFR • FFR • Hyperemia • Adenosine

KEY POINTS

• Physiologically guided revascularization improves outcomes and reduces cost.
• Current use of hyperemic indices, such as fractional flow reserve, is low.
• Hyperemia-free indices, such as instant wave-free ratio, have the potential to improve adoption by making assessment faster and easier.
• Comparison of iFR and FFR with a spectrum of invasive and noninvasive ischemia tests has demonstrated equivalent diagnostic accuracy.
• Clinical outcome studies are currently recruiting to definitively determine the role of iFR in the clinical domain.

INTRODUCTION

The appearance of a coronary stenosis on angiography relates poorly to its effect on underlying coronary flow.[1,2] This has led to the development and validation of several intracoronary indices of stenosis severity over the last 20 years.[3–8] Fractional flow reserve (FFR) is the most widely used clinical index. Its methodical validation has led to its incorporation into revascularization guidelines; however, despite this, the proportion of revascularization procedures guided by FFR is low.[9]

Recently, taking advantage of improved intracoronary wire technology and computational power, newer indices have been introduced into clinical practice.[10,11] By making stenosis assessment easier and faster, these indices aim to further increase the adoption of physiologic guided revascularization into routine clinical practice. Of these indices, instant wave-free ratio (iFR) is the most widely used alternative to FFR because it provides a measure of physiologic stenosis severity, using a standard pressure wire, and is calculated without the need of

Dr J. Davies is a consultant for Volcano Corp, and coinventor of iFR. Dr J. Davies and Dr J. Mayet have intellectual property interests in iFR Technology. Dr R. Petraco, Dr S. Sen, and Dr S. Nijjer have received travel support from Volcano Corporation and have contributed to educational events sponsored by Volcano Corporation and St. Jude Medical.

International Centre for Circulatory Health, National Heart and Lung Institute, Imperial College London, 59-61 North Wharf Road, London W2 1LA, UK

* Corresponding author.

E-mail address: sayan.sen@imperial.ac.uk

administration of powerful vasodilator agents, such as adenosine.[10,12] Its introduction has challenged the paradigms supporting the very use of FFR and justifiably has led to much debate about the need for hyperemia in stenosis assessment.[13–16]

This article assesses the data from contemporary human studies to address some of the common assumptions regarding hyperemic and baseline physiology in the context of the baseline pressure-derived index of iFR and the hyperemic index of FFR. We aim to determine if the available evidence supports the continued investigation, development, and use of baseline indices.

IS HYPEREMIA PHYSIOLOGICALLY ESSENTIAL FOR THE PRESSURE-ONLY ASSESSMENT OF A STENOSIS?

Intracoronary physiologic indices aim to determine the effect of a stenosis on blood flow within the vessel. However, measuring true volumetric blood flow is difficult, and accurate, reproducible measurements are challenging, time consuming, and largely used in the research laboratory. In contrast, pressure measurements are easier to obtain, more reproducible, and less time consuming to measure.[17] Overall this makes pressure-based indices more attractive for routine clinical use.

For a pressure-derived index to make inferences about underlying flow, intracoronary conditions need to be created where pressure and flow are proportional.[18] Under such conditions pressure can be used as a surrogate for flow, permitting assessment of the physiologic significance of the lesion using pressure alone. This circumvents the problems of measuring flow and provides a simpler, more clinically attractive tool.

The physiologic cornerstone of FFR relies on the principle that the pressure drop across a stenosis (ΔP) is proportional to flow (Q) when microvascular resistance (R) is stable (Equation 1), a condition that is achieved during the administration of hyperemic agents, such as adenosine, or alternatives, such as papaverine[18] (Equation 2).

$$\Delta P = QR \qquad (1)$$

When resistance is constant (R): $\Delta P \propto Q$ (2)

FFR is therefore highly dependent on hyperemic agents for its accurate calculation.[19] This dependence of FFR on hyperemia has been translated into the assumption that the physiologic condition requisite for pressure to be used as a surrogate to flow can only be achieved during hyperemia.[13,15,20]

However, this is in contrast to the original physiologic studies that have defined the understanding of coronary hemodynamics.[21,22] Using meticulous manual analysis of pressure-flow data, it has been demonstrated that it is indeed possible to categorize stenoses as mild, moderate, and severe without the need for hyperemia.[21] Gould[21] demonstrated that the most appropriate period for the assessment of a coronary stenosis is when intracoronary pressure is not confounded by the contraction and relaxation of the myocardium, thereby isolating a phase when the myocardium is passive and intracoronary pressure and flow velocity have an almost linear relationship. However, indices derived using such an approach had limited clinical applicability because they could only be identified from simultaneous measurement of pressure and flow velocity.[8,23]

Recently, the derivation of iFR demonstrated that it was possible to identify a phase in the cardiac cycle where the characteristic features ideal for stenosis assessment are found. The key advance was the demonstration that it was possible to automate the identification of the phase using sophisticated computational algorithms in real time on a beat-to-beat basis using the pressure wave-form alone (Fig. 1A).[10] Combining the simplicity of automation, the need to only measure pressure (rather than simultaneous pressure and flow) and absence of the need to induce hyperemia makes iFR highly attractive for routine clinical practice.[24]

Essential to the success of iFR was achieving conditions of stable microvascular resistance under resting conditions, because only under these conditions is pressure proportionate to flow. ADVISE showed that during the iFR wave-free period window the stability of resting resistance is equivalent to that achieved with adenosine-mediated hyperemia during the calculation of FFR (see Fig. 1B).[10] These findings suggested for the first time that, using contemporary phasic analysis to isolate the iFR wave-free period window, pressure can be used as a surrogate to flow under baseline conditions. In doing so ADVISE demonstrated that by using advanced computational algorithms, it was possible to obviate hyperemic agents, thereby providing a framework to challenge the underlying assumption that hyperemia is required for pressure-only stenosis assessment.

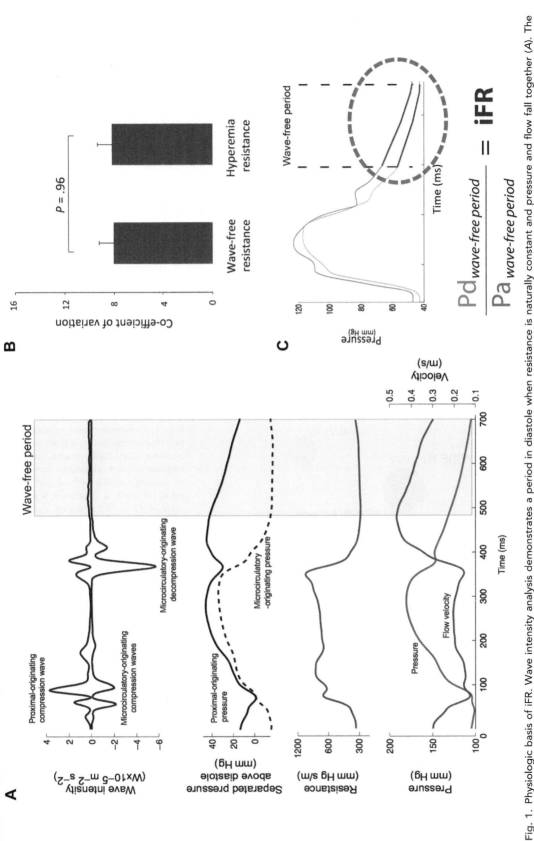

Fig. 1. Physiologic basis of iFR. Wave intensity analysis demonstrates a period in diastole when resistance is naturally constant and pressure and flow fall together (A). The stability of resistance during this "wave-free" period is equivalent to that during adenosine-mediated FFR (B). The instantaneous wave-free ratio (iFR) is calculated as the ratio of distal to proximal pressure during the diastolic wave-free period (C).

IS HYPEREMIA ESSENTIAL TO UNMASK TRUE STENOSIS SEVERITY?

Although the requisite intracoronary conditions for stenosis assessment may be available at rest the clinical utility of any resting measure of stenosis severity depends on its ability to accurately categorize a stenosis as requiring treatment or not. There are several invasive and noninvasive indices that have been used to guide revascularization decisions. The development of each invasive hyperemic index has involved a series of validation studies against other tests of ischemia. As such it is essential that any new resting index is subject to similar rigorous evaluation to assess its diagnostic performance against other invasive and noninvasive standards of ischemia.[25]

iFR has been compared with FFR in more than 3500 stenoses. The classification match to FFR-defined dichotomous categorization is approximately 80% (Fig. 2).[10,26–32] The clinical relevance of the 20% of patients where iFR and FFR disagree has been debated.[14,33–35] However, the true significance of such a figure can only be appreciated in the context of the categorization variability of FFR itself. Several studies have explored this.[26,36–39] The DEFER reproducibility study compared treatment classification of two FFR measurements across the same lesion, performed with intravenous adenosine 10 minutes apart. These data demonstrated that treatment categorization of the first FFR only matched that of the second FFR measurement in 85% of cases, with a standard deviation of the difference of two FFR measurements of 0.032.[37] There has been much debate about the accuracy of these findings because derivation of the reproducibility of FFR was made from digitization of the DEFER study data published in a Scientific Statement of the American Heart Association.[40] In addition, there has been some concern regarding the relevance of this finding to current clinical practice. This is because DEFER used first-generation pressure wires and it is conceivable that modern wires, that are less prone to drift, may have produced different results. However, despite these theoretic limitations the conclusions regarding the reproducibility of adenosine-mediated FFR were recently externally validated by a contemporary prospective study using modern pressure wires.[39] This demonstrated a standard deviation of the difference of two FFR measurements of

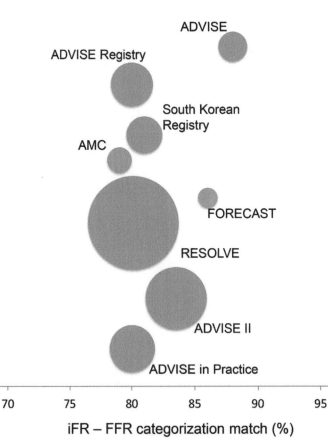

Fig. 2. Prospective and retrospective studies comparing iFR with FFR in more than 3500 lesions, using Imperial-derived algorithm (*green*) or investigator-derived algorithms (*blue*). There is a consistent agreement of iFR to FFR of approximately 80%.

iFR – FFR categorization match (%)

0.035,[39] almost identical to the value derived from the DEFER data. Additionally, Lim and colleagues[38] recently confirmed that the categorization reproducibility of adenosine-mediated FFR is 80% around the treatment threshold of 0.8. In fact, the agreement of repeated measurements of FFR seems to vary as a function of the route of adenosine administration, the type of hyperemic agent used, and the time interval between repeated measures.[38] These studies suggest that, in a typical clinical distribution of stenoses, it is unlikely that any new measure of stenosis severity will agree with FFR above a level of 80% to 85%, simply because this is the level of agreement of two adenosine-mediated FFRs. This is not just an FFR phenomenon; such measurement variability is intrinsic to any biologic measure.

Therefore, when iFR and FFR disagree how should one determine which index is more indicative of the severity of the stenosis? Several groups around the world have addressed the problem by comparing the diagnostic accuracy of iFR and FFR against the very same reference standards that were used to validate FFR itself, with the measurements of FFR and iFR being made temporally as close together as is practically feasible. Comparing iFR and FFR with these reference standards under identical conditions would provide a validation for iFR similar to that of FFR, and importantly remove the difficulties associated with the inherent variability of FFR as identified in the DEFER and other reproducibility studies. Furthermore, such analyses would provide an improved understanding of the type of patients in which iFR and FFR are likely to disagree, and potentially elicit mechanisms responsible for such disagreement. It would also allow a scientific determination of which index is more likely to indicate true stenosis severity. Such comparisons have now been performed in more than 500 lesions in five different studies using invasive and noninvasive reference standards of ischemia.[12,32,41–43] In all cases iFR was at least as accurate as FFR (Fig. 3).

In two studies in which intracoronary flow was used as part of the reference standard iFR was found to be more accurate than FFR.[33,41,42] These were the first studies to suggest that a resting index may be more accurate than a hyperemic index. A possible explanation for this was provided in a collaborative study of more than 200 lesions comparing iFR and FFR with coronary flow reserve.[42] This performed a detailed analysis of patients in which iFR and FFR disagreed. It demonstrated that when iFR and FFR disagreed, iFR was more consistent

with underlying blood flow than FFR. When iFR was normal and FFR abnormal, underling coronary flow was predominantly normal. Similarly when iFR was abnormal and FFR normal, underlying coronary flow was predominantly abnormal (Fig. 4). Most importantly the relationship between FFR and underlying coronary flow was worst (falling to 59% accuracy) in the 0.6 to 0.9 FFR range where diagnostic accuracy is absolutely critical. This finding supports other observations that have described discordance between FFR and flow of 30% to 40%, which predominately occurs in the FFR 0.6 to 0.9 range.[40] However, the new observation from the JUSTIFY-CFR analyses was that iFR agreement with underlying flow was not only better than that of FFR across the entire range, but was highly significantly better over the clinically relevant intermediate zone (0.6–0.9 FFR range). In JUSTIFY-CFR the agreement between FFR and flow in the intermediate zone fell to less than 60%. This provides a unique insight into discordance between iFR and FFR. Previously it had been assumed that the reduced agreement of iFR and FFR in the intermediate zone was caused by the lack of hyperemia during iFR. These analyses suggest that the primary source of disconcordance between iFR and FFR is an inability of FFR to adequately reflect underlying flow conditions, especially in the critical intermediate zone.

These and other results highlight the dependency of FFR on maximal hyperemia and therefore its dependency on the microvasculature, which is responsible for creating maximal hyperemia in response to the administration of hyperemic agents. The susceptibility of FFR to poorly reflect underlying flow in the coronary artery as reported by Gould and colleagues[44] varies according to the unpredictable response of the microcirculation to adenosine.[12,45] The relative independence of iFR from the microcirculation and therefore insusceptibility of iFR to this kind of error makes it potentially a more clinically attractive tool, especially in patient cohorts where the microcirculatory response to adenosine is likely to be attenuated, such as subjects with diabetes and hypertension.

IS HYPEREMIA USEFUL IN VESSELS WITH TANDEM STENOSES?

The reliance of FFR on maximal hyperemia has prevented it from being used to isolate individual stenosis severity in vessels with tandem lesions.[46] This is because when trying to assess the significance of proximal stenoses the distal

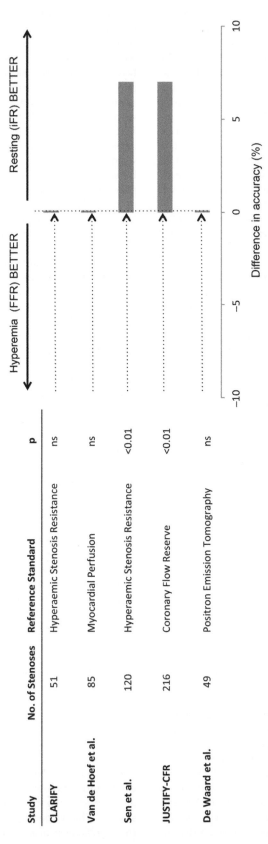

Fig. 3. Comparison of iFR and FFR with an independent measure of stenosis severity in five studies including more than 500 lesions. The administration of adenosine does not improve diagnostic accuracy. In two studies the resting index seems to be a more representative measure of the severity of the stenosis.

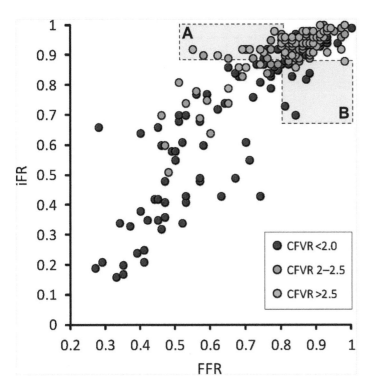

Fig. 4. When iFR and FFR disagree, iFR is more likely to agree with underlying flow. When the iFR is negative and the FFR positive the most vessels have normal flow (A). Similarly when iFR is positive and FFR negative most vessels have abnormal flow (B).

stenosis blunts hyperemic flow across the proximal lesion, therefore placement of the pressure sensor in between the two stenoses underestimates the severity of the proximal lesion (Fig. 5A). In such a scenario, when the distal lesion is treated, hyperemic flow significantly increases and as a result the FFR of the proximal vessel is significantly different (see Fig. 5B). This is circumvented in clinical practice by passing the pressure wire to the distal vessel and performing a pullback of the pressure wire during hyperemia. Once the lesion responsible for the greatest pressure drop on the pullback curve is treated the pullback is repeated to identify the next significant lesion. The assessment of multiple lesions within a single vessel using this approach requires several hyperemic pullback runs,[47] which is time consuming, adds additional expense, and most importantly is uncomfortable for patients.

Baseline indices, in contrast, are uniquely suited to the assessment of tandem lesions.[48] This is because baseline flow is maintained constant until stenosis grades of greater than 90%.[49,50] As a result iFR is able to isolate severity of a specific stenosis within a vessel with multiple lesions.[48] When the distal lesion is treated, in contrast to hyperemic flow, baseline flow is significantly less. This means that the pressure

drop across the proximal stenosis and its physiologic iFR value remains far more stable (see Fig. 5B). A recent study has systematically assessed this in patients with diffuse and tandem coronary stenoses.[46]

Although clearly circumventing a key limitation that has hampered the use of hyperemia-based indices in these patients, this also has the possibility of extending the role of physiology in interventional cardiology.[51] Rather than simply informing that a vessel is ischemic, real-time hyperemia free point-to-point calculation of iFR along the entire vessel informs where to stent to get the best hemodynamic result within a matter of seconds. Most importantly, this removes the need for multiple hyperemic pullback runs. By incorporation of real-time coregistration such an approach can be expected to significantly reduce stent length, procedural time, and costs and expand the benefits of physiologically guided revascularization to a cohort of patients that are increasingly prevalent but suboptimally served by existing hyperemic indices.

FUTURE AREAS FOR DEVELOPMENT

The studies completed so far have demonstrated that iFR and FFR agree against reference

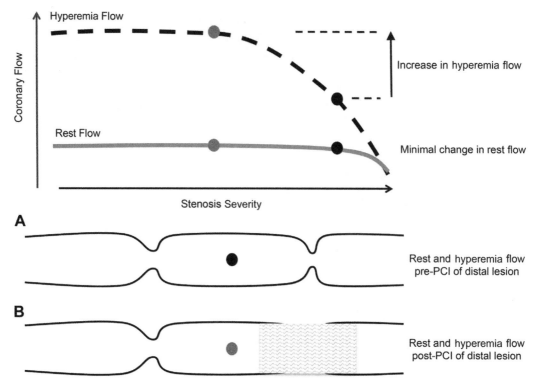

Fig. 5. How resting flow and hyperemic flow vary with stenosis severity and the impact on tandem lesion assessment. Resting flow is maintained constant until the vessel is almost subtotally occluded. In contrast, hyperemic flow declines as stenosis severity increases. Flow measured just distal to the first stenosis at rest (A) is the same as that in exactly the same position when the distal lesion has been treated (B). However, flow measured just distal to the first stenosis during hyperemia (A) is not the same as that in exactly the same position when the distal lesion has been treated (B). This means that the resting index of iFR is able to isolate the significance of the proximal lesion but the hyperemic index of FFR is unable to because treatment of the distal lesion leads to a significant increase in hyperemic flow and therefore change in FFR. PCI, percutaneous coronary intervention.

standards in most cases. When they disagree it seems that the response of the microcirculation to hyperemic drug administration is the discriminating factor. Although iFR, by definition, is not dependent on a response of the microvasculature to a drug, FFR is heavily dependent on microvascular response to hyperemic agents.[42] This suggests that in conditions where the microvasculature response to adenosine is unreliable, such as diabetes, hypertension, and renal impairment, a more microcirculatory independent index, such as iFR, could be more informative.

The previous discussion does not negate the outcome data associated with FFR.[52,53] Rather it highlights the potential of resting indices to circumvent some of the limitations of hyperemia-dependent indices, such as FFR. Although the previous data point to equivalence of iFR to FFR in determining stenosis severity (even hinting at possible superiority of the resting index) its clinical role will ultimately be defined by large clinical outcome studies. Two randomized prospective studies comparing outcomes of iFR-guided revascularization with FFR-guided revascularization are currently recruiting (DEFINE-FLAIR [NCT02053038, 2500 patients] and iFR-Swedeheart [NCT02166736, 2000 patients]). These global physiologic studies are the largest studies in coronary physiology to date (Fig. 6). Combined they will provide a unique insight into clinical use of physiologically guided revascularization in more than 4500 patients, and more than 7500 stenoses, and will provide clinical outcome data to validate the use of iFR and thereby define the clinical need for hyperemia in this domain. In the interim, iFR has also been adopted as the first-line physiologic assessment in other major clinical trials. Both SYNTAX II (NCT02015832) and PROSPECT II (NCT02171065) use iFR. Outcome data from these studies will further define the role of iFR in routine clinical practice.

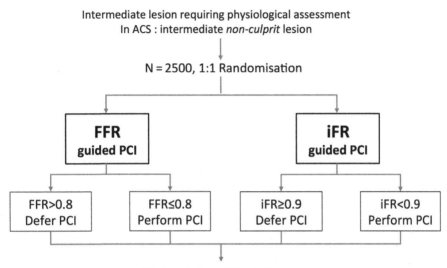

DEFINE FLAIR

Functional Lesion Assessment of Intermediate stenosis to guide Revascularisation

Intermediate lesion requiring physiological assessment
In ACS : intermediate *non-culprit* lesion

N = 2500, 1:1 Randomisation

| **FFR** guided PCI | **iFR** guided PCI |

| FFR>0.8 Defer PCI | FFR≤0.8 Perform PCI | iFR≥0.9 Defer PCI | iFR<0.9 Perform PCI |

30 day, 1, 2 and 5yr follow-up

Fig. 6. Design of the DEFINE FLAIR study. DEFINE FLAIR is a prospective randomized study to compare the clinical outcomes of an iFR-based revascularization strategy with that of an FFR-based strategy. The primary end point is a composite of death, myocardial infarction, and unplanned revascularization.

SUMMARY

There has been extensive debate in the literature regarding the need for hyperemia in stenosis assessment. The potential for resting indices, in particular iFR, has been debated on physiologic and diagnostic grounds, driving studies investigating its potential. Contrary to initial conjecture, objective scientific assessment has demonstrated that the resting index of iFR is based on sound physiology, has equivalent diagnostic accuracy to FFR, and in certain situations may be more accurate than its hyperemic counterpart. The studies to date provide a strong argument for continued investigation and validation of resting indices. Ultimately their clinical role will be established by large clinical trials but for the moment there is certainly ample evidence to question the need for hyperemia.

ACKNOWLEDGMENTS

The authors acknowledge the support of the NIHR Biomedical Research Center based at Imperial College Healthcare National Health Service (NHS) Trust and Imperial College London. The views expressed are those of the author and not necessarily those of the NHS, the NIHR, or the Department of Health. S.S. Nijjer (G1100443) and S. Sen (G1000357) are Medical Research Council fellows. Dr R. Petraco (FS/11/46/28861), and Dr J. Davies (FS/05/006) are British Heart Foundation fellows.

REFERENCES

1. Kern MJ. Seeing and not believing: understanding the visual-functional mismatch between angiography and FFR. Catheter Cardiovasc Interv 2014;84:414–5.
2. Tonino PA, Fearon WF, De Bruyne B, et al. Angiographic versus functional severity of coronary artery stenoses in the FAME study fractional flow reserve versus angiography in multivessel evaluation. J Am Coll Cardiol 2010;55:2816–21.
3. Meuwissen M, Siebes M, Spaan JA, et al. Rationale of combined intracoronary pressure and flow velocity measurements. Z Kardiol 2002; 91(Suppl 3):108–12.
4. Meuwissen M, Chamuleau SAJ, Siebes M, et al. The prognostic value of combined intracoronary pressure and blood flow velocity measurements after deferral of percutaneous coronary intervention. Catheter Cardiovasc Interv 2008;71:291–7.
5. Bruyne BD, Baudhuin T, Melin JA, et al. Coronary flow reserve calculated from pressure measurements in humans. Validation with positron emission tomography. Circulation 1994;89:1013–22.
6. Bech GJ, De Bruyne B, Akasaka T, et al. Coronary pressure and FFR predict long-term outcome after PTCA. Int J Cardiovasc Intervent 2001;4:67–76.

7. Pijls NH, De Bruyne B, Peels K, et al. Measurement of fractional flow reserve to assess the functional severity of coronary-artery stenoses. N Engl J Med 1996;334:1703–8.

8. Marques KM, van Eenige MJ, Spruijt HJ, et al. The diastolic flow velocity-pressure gradient relation and dpv50 to assess the hemodynamic significance of coronary stenoses. Am J Physiol Heart Circ Physiol 2006;291:H2630–5.

9. Kleiman NS. Bringing it all together: integration of physiology with anatomy during cardiac catheterization. J Am Coll Cardiol 2011;58:1219–21.

10. Sen S, Escaned J, Malik IS, et al. Development and validation of a new adenosine-independent index of stenosis severity from coronary wave–intensity analysis. J Am Coll Cardiol 2012;59:1392–402.

11. van de Hoef TP, Nolte F, Damman P, et al. Diagnostic accuracy of combined intracoronary pressure and flow velocity information during baseline conditions: adenosine-free assessment of functional coronary lesion severity. Circ Cardiovasc Interv 2012;5(4):508–14.

12. Sen S, Asrress KN, Nijjer S, et al. Diagnostic classification of the instantaneous wave-free ratio is equivalent to fractional flow reserve and is not improved with adenosine administration: results of clarify (classification accuracy of pressure-only ratios against indices using flow study). J Am Coll Cardiol 2013;61:1409–20.

13. Pijls NH, Van 't Veer M, Oldroyd KG, et al. Instantaneous wave-free ratio or fractional flow reserve without hyperemianovelty or nonsense? J Am Coll Cardiol 2012;59:1916–7.

14. Rudzinski W, Waller AH, Kaluski E. Instantaneous wave-free ratio and fractional flow reserve: close, but not close enough! J Am Coll Cardiol 2012;59:1915–6 [author reply: 1917–8].

15. Finet G, Rioufol G. A new adenosine-independent index of stenosis severity: why would one assess a coronary stenosis differently? J Am Coll Cardiol 2012;59:1915 [author reply: 1917–8].

16. Sen S, Escaned J, Francis D, et al. Reply. J Am Coll Cardiol 2012;59:1917–8.

17. De Bruyne B, Bartunek J, Sys SU, et al. Simultaneous coronary pressure and flow velocity measurements in humans. Feasibility, reproducibility, and hemodynamic dependence of coronary flow velocity reserve, hyperemic flow versus pressure slope index, and fractional flow reserve. Circulation 1996;94:1842–9.

18. Pijls NH, van Son JA, Kirkeeide RL, et al. Experimental basis of determining maximum coronary, myocardial, and collateral blood flow by pressure measurements for assessing functional stenosis severity before and after percutaneous transluminal coronary angioplasty. Circulation 1993;87: 1354–67.

19. Pijls NHJ, Tonino PAL. The crux of maximum hyperemia: the last remaining barrier for routine use of fractional flow reserve. JACC Cardiovasc Interv 2011;4:1093–5.

20. Samady H, Gogas BD. Does flow during rest and relaxation suffice? J Am Coll Cardiol 2013;61: 1436–9.

21. Gould KL. Pressure-flow characteristics of coronary stenoses in unsedated dogs at rest and during coronary vasodilation. Circ Res 1978;43:242–53.

22. Gould KL, Lipscomb K, Calvert C. Compensatory changes of the distal coronary vascular bed during progressive coronary constriction. Circulation 1975; 51:1085–94.

23. Marques KM, Spruijt HJ, Boer C, et al. The diastolic flow-pressure gradient relation in coronary stenoses in humans. J Am Coll Cardiol 2002;39:1630–6.

24. Kern MJ. An adenosine-independent index of stenosis severity from coronary wave-intensity analysis: a new paradigm in coronary physiology for the cath lab? J Am Coll Cardiol 2012;59:1403–5.

25. Christou MA, Siontis GC, Katritsis DG, et al. Meta-analysis of fractional flow reserve versus quantitative coronary angiography and noninvasive imaging for evaluation of myocardial ischemia. Am J Cardiol 2007;99:450–6.

26. Petraco R, Escaned J, Sen S, et al. Classification performance of instantaneous wave-free ratio (iFR) and fractional flow reserve in a clinical population of intermediate coronary stenoses: results of the ADVISE registry. EuroIntervention 2013;9:91–101.

27. Park JJ, Petraco R, Nam CW, et al. Clinical validation of the resting pressure parameters in the assessment of functionally significant coronary stenosis; results of an independent, blinded comparison with fractional flow reserve. Int J Cardiol 2013; 168:4070–5.

28. Escaned J, Echavarría-Pinto M, Garcia-Garcia HM, et al. Prospective Assessment of the Diagnostic Accuracy of Instantaneous Wave-Free Ratio to Assess Coronary Stenosis Relevance: Results of ADVISE II International, Multicenter Study (ADenosine Vasodilator Independent Stenosis Evaluation II). JACC Cardiovasc Interv 2015;8(6):824–33.

29. Indolfi C, Mongiardo A, Spaccarotella C, et al. The instantaneous wave-free ratio (iFR) for evaluation of non-culprit lesions in patients with acute coronary syndrome and multivessel disease. Int J Cardiol 2014;178C:46–54.

30. Petraco R, Al-Lamee R, Gotberg M, et al. Real-time use of instantaneous wave-free ratio: results of the ADVISE in-practice: an international, multicenter evaluation of instantaneous wave-free ratio in clinical practice. Am Heart J 2014;168:739–48.

31. Jeremias A, Maehara A, Généreux P, et al. Multicenter core laboratory comparison of the instantaneous wave-free ratio and resting Pd/Pa with

fractional flow reserve: the RESOLVE study. J Am Coll Cardiol 2014;63:1253–61.

32. Van de Hoef TP, Meuwissen M, Escaned J, et al. Head-to-head comparison of basal stenosis resistance index, instantaneous wave-free ratio, and fractional flow reserve: diagnostic accuracy for stenosis-specific myocardial ischaemia. EuroIntervention 2014. [Epub ahead of print].

33. Johnson NP, Kirkeeide RL, Asrress KN, et al. Does the instantaneous wave-free ratio approximate the fractional flow reserve? J Am Coll Cardiol 2013;61:1428–35.

34. Petraco R, Escaned J, Sen S, et al. How high can "accuracy" be for iFR (or IVUS, or SPECT, or OCT...) if using fractional flow reserve as the gold standard? EuroIntervention 2013;9:770–2.

35. Petraco R, Escaned J, Nijjer S, et al. Reply: fractional flow reserve: a good or a gold standard? JACC Cardiovasc Interv 2014;7:228–9.

36. Bech GJ, Bruyne BD, Pijls NH, et al. Fractional flow reserve to determine the appropriateness of angioplasty in moderate coronary stenosis a randomized trial. Circulation 2001;103:2928–34.

37. Petraco R, Sen S, Nijjer S, et al. Fractional flow reserve-guided revascularization: practical implications of a diagnostic gray zone and measurement variability on clinical decisions. JACC Cardiovasc Interv 2013;6(3):222–5.

38. Lim WH, Koo BK, Nam CW, et al. Variability of fractional flow reserve according to the methods of hyperemia induction. Catheter Cardiovasc Interv 2015;85(6):970–6.

39. Gaur S, Bezerra HG, Lassen JF, et al. Fractional flow reserve derived from coronary CT angiography: variation of repeated analyses. J Cardiovasc Comput Tomogr 2014;8:307–14.

40. Kern MJ, Lerman A, Bech J-W, et al. Physiological assessment of coronary artery disease in the cardiac catheterization laboratory a scientific statement from the American Heart Association Committee on Diagnostic and Interventional Cardiac Catheterization, Council on Clinical Cardiology. Circulation 2006;114:1321–41.

41. Sen S, Nijjer S, Petraco R, et al. Instantaneous wave-free ratio: numerically different, but diagnostically superior to FFR? is lower always better? J Am Coll Cardiol 2013;62:566.

42. Petraco R, van de Hoef TP, Nijjer S, et al. Baseline instantaneous wave-free ratio as a pressure-only estimation of underlying coronary flow reserve: results of the JUSTIFY-CFR Study (Joined Coronary Pressure and Flow Analysis to Determine Diagnostic Characteristics of Basal and Hyperemic Indices of Functional Lesion Severity-Coronary Flow Reserve). Circ Cardiovasc Interv 2014;7:492–502.

43. De Waard G, Danad I, da Cunha RP, et al. Hyperemic FFR and baseline iFR have an equivalent diagnostic accuracy when compared to myocardial blood flow quantified by $H_2^{15}O$ pet perfusion imaging. J Am Coll Cardiol 2014;63:A1692.

44. Gould KL, Johnson NP, Bateman TM, et al. Anatomic versus physiologic assessment of coronary artery disease. Role of coronary flow reserve, fractional flow reserve, and positron emission tomography imaging in revascularization decision-making. J Am Coll Cardiol 2013;62:1639–53.

45. Seto AH, Tehrani DM, Bharmal MI, et al. Variations of coronary hemodynamic responses to intravenous adenosine infusion: implications for fractional flow reserve measurements. Catheter Cardiovasc Interv 2014;84:416–25.

46. Bruyne BD, Pijls NH, Heyndrickx GR, et al. Pressure-derived fractional flow reserve to assess serial epicardial stenoses theoretical basis and animal validation. Circulation 2000;101:1840–7.

47. Kim H-L, Koo B-K, Nam C-W, et al. Clinical and physiological outcomes of fractional flow reserve-guided percutaneous coronary intervention in patients with serial stenoses within one coronary artery. JACC Cardiovasc Interv 2012;5:1013–8.

48. Nijjer SS, Sen S, Petraco R, et al. Pre-angioplasty instantaneous wave-free ratio (iFR) pullback provides virtual intervention and predicts hemodynamic outcome for serial lesions and diffuse coronary artery disease. JACC Cardiovasc Interv 2014;7(12):1386–96.

49. Gould KL, Lipscomb K, Hamilton GW. Physiologic basis for assessing critical coronary stenosis: instantaneous flow response and regional distribution during coronary hyperemia as measures of coronary flow reserve. Am J Cardiol 1974;33:87–94.

50. Gould KL, Kelley KO. Physiological significance of coronary flow velocity and changing stenosis geometry during coronary vasodilation in awake dogs. Circ Res 1982;50:695–704.

51. Piek JJ, van de Hoef TP. Pre-angioplasty instantaneous wave-free ratio pullback and virtual revascularization: the pressure wire as a crystal ball. JACC Cardiovasc Interv 2014;7:1397–9.

52. Tonino PA, De Bruyne B, Pijls NH, et al. Fractional flow reserve versus angiography for guiding percutaneous coronary intervention. N Engl J Med 2009;360:213–24.

53. De Bruyne B, Fearon WF, Pijls NH, et al. Fractional flow reserve-guided PCI for stable coronary artery disease. N Engl J Med 2014;371:1208–17.

Fractional Flow Reserve for the Evaluation of Tandem and Bifurcation Lesions, Left Main, and Acute Coronary Syndromes

Jaya Mallidi, MD, MHS, Amir Lotfi, MD, FSCAI*

KEYWORDS

- FFR • Tandem lesions • Bifurcation lesions • Left main disease • ACS

KEY POINTS

- Subjects with tandem lesions, bifurcation lesions, left main disease, and acute coronary syndrome are not included in trials supporting fractional flow reserve (FFR)-guided revascularization.
- Assessment and interpretation of FFR in these clinical scenarios is technically challenging due to the unique changes in flow hemodynamics in each of these situations.
- The existing literature supports the safety of using FFR to guide revascularization in these situations; however, the evidence is limited and further research is warranted.

INTRODUCTION

Fractional flow reserve (FFR) is a well-established adjunctive tool to coronary angiography to evaluate the physiologic significance of intermediate coronary stenosis (40%–70%). FFR is defined as the ratio of myocardial blood flow in a coronary artery in the presence of an epicardial stenosis compared with the hypothetical blood flow in the same coronary artery without stenosis in conditions of maximum achievable hyperemia.[1] FFR of a single coronary artery lesion can be measured as the ratio of the mean distal coronary artery pressure (P_d) to the mean aortic pressure (P_a) during maximum hyperemia.

Several multicenter, randomized trials support FFR-guided revascularization in subjects with single or multivessel stable coronary artery disease.[2–4] In everyday practice, scenarios such as tandem and bifurcation lesions, left main coronary artery (LMCA) disease, and acute coronary syndrome (ACS) are encountered. The literature supporting the use of FFR for clinical decision-making in these situations is limited. This article reviews the technical aspects and challenges in assessing FFR and using it to guide revascularization in these situations.

FRACTIONAL FLOW RESERVE IN TANDEM LESIONS

Tandem lesions are defined as 2 lesions separated by an intervening angiographically normal segment. With tandem lesions the presence of a distal lesion decreases the hyperemic flow through the proximal lesion, changing the relative severity of the proximal lesion.[5] Hence, in serial lesions, FFR calculated by the ratio of P_d to P_a for a proximal lesion in the presence of a distal stenosis is not the same as the FFR calculated for the same lesion after the relief of distal stenosis and vice versa.

Conflict of Interest: None.

Division of Cardiology, Baystate Medical Center, Tufts University, 759 Chestnut Street, Springfield, MA 01199, USA

* Corresponding author.

E-mail address: amir.lotfi@bhs.org

Intervent Cardiol Clin 4 (2015) 471–480

http://dx.doi.org/10.1016/j.iccl.2015.06.007

De Bruyne and colleagues[5] developed theoretic equations from animal models to predict FFR of each serial stenosis as if the other stenosis was not present. The FFR of each serial stenosis can be calculated separately by obtaining the proximal aortic pressure (P_a), pressure beyond the distal stenosis (P_d), pressure between the 2 stenoses (P_m) and the coronary wedge pressure (P_w) during the period of maximum hyperemia.[5] These equations were subsequently validated by Pijls and colleagues[6] in human subjects (Fig. 1). True FFR (FFR $_{true}$) of each stenosis measured after stenting of the other stenosis when compared with predicted FFR (FFR$_{pred}$) derived from the equations before the intervention were closely correlated ($r = 0.92$).[6]

There are some practical limitations in using the equations described in Fig. 1. P_w can only be obtained during balloon coronary occlusion. Therefore, the commitment to the intervention of the lesion is made by the time it is measured. P_w represents the degree of myocardial blood flow that is composed of collaterals. It is different in each patient depending on the extent of developed collateral circulation and hence, should be measured in every patient.[6] Also, these equations are only applicable to serial lesions without an intervening arterial side branch, which provides a low resistance to the flow of blood. The quantification of FFR in this situation is complex and requires the development of computational fluid dynamic equations accounting for myocardial mass supplied by each side branch.[7,8]

In a study involving 131 subjects from 2 large Korean centers, Kim and colleagues[9] described the long-term outcomes of using FFR measured by pullback pressure tracings to guide revascularization in subjects with tandem lesions in a single coronary vessel. In this study, the lesion that caused the largest pressure step-up was treated first (primary target lesion). The second stenosis was treated only if the FFR was significant after stenting the primary target lesion. In 61% of the lesions, revascularization was deferred based on the FFR. There were no events related to deferred lesions, suggesting that FFR-guided revascularization using pullback pressure tracings in tandem lesions is safe and effective.[9] Using in vitro computational flow dynamic models in tandem lesions, Park and colleagues[10] also validated that FFR gradient (delta FFR) across a stenosis during pressure wire pullback is a surrogate estimate of relative functional severity of that lesion. Hence, the stenosis with the largest delta FFR is treated first and the FFR across the second lesion is rechecked again. This is a more practical approach for deciding which lesion to treat first and does not require the measurement of P_w.

The following are the steps involved in repetitive pressure pullback technique of assessing tandem lesions (Fig. 2):

1. The pressure wire is advanced into the target vessel distal to the most distal stenosis.
2. During period of maximum hyperemia, the pressure step-up across each individual lesion is measured by pulling back the pressure wire from the distal coronary artery to the ostium.

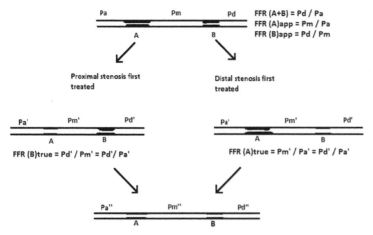

Fig. 1. Treatment sequence in patients with serial stenosis in the same coronary artery. FFR (A)$_{true}$ and FFR (B)$_{true}$, measured after complete elimination of stenosis A and B were closely correlated to the FFR (A)$_{predicted}$ and FFR (B)$_{predicted}$ from the equations. (*From* Pijls NH, De Bruyne B, Bech GJ, et al. Coronary pressure measurement to assess the hemodynamic significance of serial stenoses within one coronary artery: validation in humans. Circulation 2000;102(19):2372; with permission.)

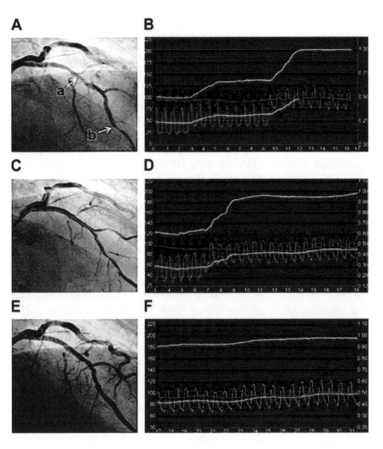

A **B**

C **D**

E **F**

Fig. 2. Representative case of FFR with pullback pressure tracing-guided PCI. (*A, B*) Tandem lesions (*a* and *b*) were observed in the left anterior descending artery. Because measured FFR was 0.48, pullback pressure tracing while monitoring intracoronary pressure (*green line*), aortic pressure (*red line*), and FFR (*yellow line*) was performed. Two step-ups were observed. (*B*) Apparent FFR of lesions a and b were 0.67 (ratio of pressures 60:90) and 0.75 (ratio of pressures 45:60), respectively. Lesion a was stented first due to the larger step-up (30 mm Hg). (*C, D*) After stenting lesion a (*C*), pullback pressure tracings were performed again. Intracoronary pressure step-up across lesion b was 20 mm Hg, and FFR $_{true}$ was 0.73. (*E, F*) After stenting both lesions, FFR was 0.85. (*From* Kim HL, Koo BK, Nam CW, et al. Clinical and physiologic outcomes of fractional flow reserve-guided percutaneous coronary intervention in patients with serial stenoses within one coronary artery. JACC Cardiovasc Interv 2012;5(10):1015; with permission.)

3. The lesion across which the maximum pressure step-up is recorded is dilated and stented first.
4. After stenting 1 lesion, a pull-back pressure recording at maximum hyperemia is again recorded. The second stenosis is then dilated and stented if the FFR is significant.

In summary, in patients with stable coronary artery disease, found to have tandem coronary lesions, FFR-guided revascularization is safe. Repetitive pressure pullback technique is a practically useful technique in finding out the lesion with largest pressure step-up, treating the primary lesion first, and subsequently determining the significance of the second stenosis.

FRACTIONAL FLOW RESERVE IN OSTIAL OR BIFURCATION LESIONS

A bifurcation lesion is defined as, "a coronary artery narrowing occuring adjacent to, and/ or involving the origin of a significant side branch."[11] The stenosis at the origin of the side branch could be either due to presence of plaque before the intervention or could be the result of jailing the side branch during stenting of the main vessel. The decision whether to intervene and the technique to be used for side branch intervention can be challenging for the following reasons.

Difficulty in Angiographic or Anatomic Evaluation

Angiographic evaluation of bifurcation lesions is difficult and not accurate because of complex geometry, angulation, vessel overlap, image foreshortening, and eccentricity of the plaque in the ostial side branches.[12] Also, in jailed side branches, the mechanism of stenosis is complex, involving shifting of the plaque into the carina, spasm, and presence of stent struts.[12] The functional severity of the jailed side branches is often overestimated by angiography.[13] Anatomic evaluation using intravascular ultrasound (IVUS) or optical computed tomography is also not helpful because it is technically challenging and there are no validated criteria for side branch interventions.[14]

Outcomes of Percutaneous Coronary Intervention of Ostial or Bifurcation Lesions Are Poor

Percutaneous coronary interventions (PCIs) of bifurcation lesions are associated with higher rates of major cardiovascular events compared with nonbifurcation lesions.[15–17] The optimal treatment of these lesions is controversial. In the jailed side branches, balloon angioplasty or no intervention might be superior in terms of long-term clinical outcomes compared with stenting.[16] In a recent computational flow dynamics study, Williams and colleagues[18] demonstrated that intervention of nonfunctionally significant side branch lesions will not improve the local flow conditions in bifurcation lesions.

In patients with true bifurcation lesions and long side branches, the optimal stenting technique is not well established. Stenting of the main vessel followed by provisional stenting of the side branch is currently the preferred approach compared with a complex strategy involving the deployment of stents in both vessels (**Fig. 3**).[19] However, in bifurcation lesions with large side branches, higher rates of repeat interventions were seen in the simple compared with the complex strategy.[19] Given the difficulty in accurately assessing the severity of bifurcation lesions by angiography, the technical complexity of the intervention, and subsequent poor outcomes after a complex intervention, it is important to define the functional significance of the side branch lesions before intervention.

Koo and colleagues[20] described the long-term outcomes of FFR-guided jailed side branch interventions in a study involving 220 subjects. This was a nonrandomized study with 2 groups of subjects: FFR-guided side branch intervention and conventional group. There was no difference in the cardiac event rates between these groups (4.6 vs 3.7%, $P = .7$).[20] However, the number of complex side branch interventions was significantly lower in the FFR-guided group (30% vs 45%, $P = .03$).[20] This suggests that FFR-guided intervention of the jailed side branches is safe and may be helpful in reducing the number of unnecessary interventions. The measurement of FFR after side branch angioplasty or stenting to optimize the results of coronary stenting has not been proven helpful so far.[21]

The following are some of the practical issues encountered when trying to determine the FFR of the jailed side branch after main vessel stenting:

1. To measure the FFR of the jailed side branch, the pressure wire should be passed through the stent struts of the main vessel. Care should be taken not to jail the pressure wire itself against the stent struts.[22]
2. The pressure wire has decreased torquability and flexibility compared with a workhorse wire. Hence, it can be difficult to engage the side branch. In these cases, the workhorse guide wire can be used to engage the side

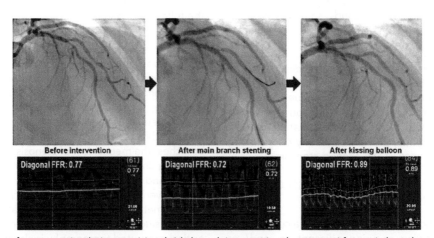

Fig. 3. Use of pressure wire during provisional side branch interventional strategy. After main branch stent implantation, side branch ostial lesion has become functionally significant. After kissing balloon inflation, FFR has increased to 0.89 despite angiographically significant residual stenosis. (*From* Koo BK, De Bruyne B. FFR in bifurcation stenting: what have we learned? EuroIntervention 2010;6 Suppl J:J96; with permission.)

branch lesion, and subsequently exchange it for an FFR wire with the help of an exchange microcatheter.[23]

3. The distal side branch disease as well as the proximal main branch disease should be taken into account when assessing the FFR of the ostial side branch lesion.

In summary, angiography often overestimates the functional significance of ostial or bifurcation lesions. Percutaneous intervention of these lesions is complex and associated with poor outcomes. To date, there are no large-scale randomized trials advocating the use of FFR-guided intervention in all bifurcation lesions. In small side branches in which clinically revascularization is not indicated, FFR need not be performed. However, in moderately sized side branches, deferral of revascularization based on FFR is safe and helps in reducing unnecessary complex interventions.

FRACTIONAL FLOW RESERVE IN LEFT MAIN CORONARY ARTERY DISEASE

Significant LMCA stenosis is angiographically defined as greater than 50% luminal narrowing. It is important to accurately assess the severity of LMCA disease because the mortality benefit of revascularization in significant unprotected LMCA disease is well established.[24] However, visual assessment of LMCA stenosis by angiography alone is challenging and is associated with significant interobserver variability given its short length, lack of a distinct reference segment, presence of overlapping branches, contrast streaming, and reverse tapering often seen at the ostium.[25] Also, the physiologic significance of the lesion cannot be assessed based on angiography alone.[26]

To date, there are no large-scale randomized trials comparing FFR-guided and angiography-guided revascularization strategies in unprotected LMCA disease. Table 1 shows all the prospective cohort studies that evaluated revascularization of LMCA stenosis based on FFR. In one of the largest studies, by Hamilos and colleagues,[27] involving 213 subjects with intermediate LMCA stenosis, revascularization was deferred if FFR was greater than 0.80. The 5-year survival estimates and event-free survival estimates were similar in the medically treated as well as revascularized groups.[27] On a similar note, in the study by Courtis and colleagues,[28] the incidence of major cardiovascular events related to LMCA stenosis were similar in both groups.

The following are important caveats that need to be considered when assessing FFR in LMCA stenosis:

1. Significant LMCA stenosis is often associated with downstream stenosis in either the left anterior descending or left circumflex artery, which may overestimate the FFR measurement.[29] However, a recent study done in animal models by Yong and colleagues[30] demonstrated that FFR of LMCA stenosis can be safely measured if the pressure wire is placed in the nonstenosed downstream vessel. Clinically relevant effect on FFR will occur only if there is severe proximal stenosis in the other epicardial vessel.[30] Because downstream disease usually results in overestimation of FFR, a value less than 0.75 will accurately identify significant LMCA disease requiring revascularization and FFR value of greater than 0.85 indicates that LMCA disease is not functionally significant despite presence of downstream disease.[30]

2. If the FFR is between 0.80 and 0.85, complementary use of IVUS is advocated to assess LMCA severity.[25] An IVUS minimal lumen diameter of 2.8 mm and minimal lumen area of 5.9 mm^2 were shown to predict the physiologic significance of LMCA stenosis.[31]

3. Sometimes, because of the individualistic variation in hyperemic response, higher doses of adenosine might have to be used to achieve the maximum hyperemic response.[32]

Despite these caveats in measuring FFR in LMCA stenosis, based on the limited evidence from all the available studies, deferral of revascularization based on FFR results seems to be safe. The current expert consensus guidelines on the use of FFR endorse a cut-off value of 0.75 to 0.80 to guide clinical decision-making regarding revascularization in intermediate LMCA stenosis.[33]

FRACTIONAL FLOW RESERVE IN ACUTE CORONARY SYNDROMES

The use of FFR in ACS is not well-established. The pathophysiology of ACS involves dynamic changes in the microvascular resistance depending on several factors, such as the extent and duration of ischemia, changes in systemic and local vasoconstrictors, downstream embolization of thrombus into the microvasculature, acute changes in filling pressure, and wall stress.[34] These changes occur within the first few hours to days after the acute event. The microvascular resistance is, therefore, not constant during

Table 1
Studies using fractional flow reserve to guide unprotected left main intervention

Study	Number of Subjects	Defining iLM (%)	FFR Cut-off	Follow-up (mo)	Defer	Revascularization of LM	Survival Defer (%)	Survival Revascularization (%)	RR CI (95% CI)
Bech et al	54	40–60	0.75	29 ± 15	24	30 CABG	100	97	0.80 (0.05–12.13)
Jimenez Navarro et al	27	30–50	0.75	26 ± 12	20	7 CABG	100	86	7.87 (0.35–173.98)
Legutko et al	38	30–60	0.75	24 (12–36)	20	12 CABG, 5 PCI, 1 OMT	100	89	5.526 (0.28–107.96)
Suemaru et al	15	25–75	0.75	32.5 ± 9.7	8	7 CABG	100	100	Excluded
Lindstaedt et al[a]	51	40–80	0.75–0.80	29 ± 16	24	27 CABG	100	81	8.03 (0.45–141.94)
Courtis et al[b]	142	30–60	0.75	14 ± 11	82	54 CABG, 6 PCI	96	95	1.36 (0.28–6.53)
Hamilos et al[a]	213	30–70	<0.8	36 (6–99)	138	75 CABG	89.8	85.4	1.84 (0.67–5.04)
Total	540	—	—	—	316	224	96	90	2.28 (1.12–4.60)[c]

Abbreviations: CABG, coronary artery bypass grafting; CI, confidence interval; iLM, intermediate left main; LM, left main; OMT, optimal medical therapy; RR, relative risk.
[a] Route of adenosine: intravenous.
[b] Route of adenosine: intracoronary.
[c] Heterogeneity Chi^2 = 2.85 (df = 5), P = .723 I^2 (variation in RR attributable to heterogeneity) = 0.0%. Test of RR = 1, z = 2.30, P = .022.

From Lotfi A, Jeremias A, Fearon WF, et al. Expert consensus statement on the use of fractional flow reserve, intravascular ultrasound, and optical coherence tomography: a consensus statement of the society of cardiovascular angiography and interventions. Catheter Cardiovasc Interv 2014;83(4):512; with permission.

ACS. Maximum hyperemia is difficult to achieve with dynamic microvascular resistance and dysfunction. Due to increased microvascular resistance, FFR is often overestimated in these situations.[35] Hence, FFR measurement in ACS may not be reliable, especially in the culprit vessel in the acute phase of ACS. It is neither practical nor useful to measure FFR in a culprit vessel in acute ST elevation myocardial infarction (STEMI). However, recent clinical studies show that FFR might be a valid concept in other clinical scenarios of ACS in which the changes in microvascular resistance are not as profound as in acute STEMI.[36–39]

Fractional Flow Reserve in Chronic Myocardial Infarction

The dynamic changes in microvascular resistance seen during the acute phase after myocardial infarction are not present after several days. A high FFR in the culprit vessel after several days represents the small amount of viable myocardium that is supplied by the vessel.[36] Hence, it provides useful information regarding the benefit of revascularization in chronic myocardial infarction. De Bruyne and colleagues[36] compared FFR values with single photon emission photography (SPECT) imaging before and after PCI in 57 subjects who sustained an old myocardial infarction. An FFR cut-off value of 0.75 was noted to have a sensitivity and specificity of 82% and 87%, respectively, to detect reversible ischemia in regions of partially infarcted territories.[36] In a study by Samady and colleagues[40] involving 48 subjects, similar findings were noted. FFR cut-off value of 0.78 in an infarct-related artery accurately identified reversibility on noninvasive testing. Thus, several days after a myocardial infarction, measurement of FFR can accurately identify the presence of ischemia and identify patients who would most benefit from revascularization.

Fractional Flow Reserve of Nonculprit Vessel in ST Elevation Myocardial Infarction

Multivessel disease is present in 40% to 65% of STEMI patients undergoing PCI and is associated with worse clinical outcomes.[41] The current STEMI guidelines recommend treating only the culprit vessel at the time of primary PCI.[42] The management of nonculprit vessels in terms of defining the hemodynamic significance and the timing of subsequent revascularization if necessary is controversial.[43,44]

Ntalianis and colleagues[45] showed that the severity of nonculprit vessel stenosis can reliably be assessed by FFR in the acute phase of ACS

even in STEMI subjects. In 75 subjects with STEMI, FFR value of the nonculprit vessel did not change between the acute phase and follow-up at 35 days.[45] Thus, measuring FFR in the acute phase of myocardial infarction in the nonculprit vessel may be helpful in risk stratification and decrease the need for additional noninvasive testing to detect residual myocardial ischemia. Large-scale randomized trials to assess the long-term clinical outcomes in an FFR-guided revascularization strategy in nonculprit vessels in STEMI are still ongoing at this time (NCT01399736).

Fractional Flow Reserve in Non–ST Elevation Myocardial Infarction

A significant portion of patients presenting with non-STEMI (NSTEMI) have multivessel disease. Because changes in microvascular resistance are not as profound as in STEMI patients, FFR can be used for the evaluation of culprit as well as nonculprit vessels in NSTEMI.

In a study to evaluate the value of FFR in NSTEMI, Leesar and colleagues[37] randomized 71 subjects who had recent unstable angina or NSTEMI with an intermediate single vessel disease to either stress perfusion scintigraphy or FFR-guided revascularization after stabilization and medical therapy for 48 hours. There was no difference between the groups in long-term outcomes.[37] The use of FFR was associated with marked reduction in the duration and cost of hospitalization.[37] This trial was conducted in an era when routine early invasive management was not the advocated approach in NSTEMI.

In a subgroup analysis of 328 NSTEMI subjects from the Fractional flow reserve versus Angiography for Multivessel Evaluation (FAME) study,[3] Sels and colleagues[38] showed that the benefits of FFR-guided PCI in unstable angina and NSTEMI were similar to those in subjects with stable angina. The total number of stents placed was reduced in the FFR-guided group compared with angiographic group (1.9 + 1.5 vs 2.9 + 1.1, $P<.01$).[38] The absolute risk reduction in major cardiovascular events was noted to be 5.1%, comparable with 3.7% in subjects with stable angina.[38]

Fractional Flow Reserve versus Angiography in Guiding Management to Optimize Outcomes in Non–ST-Segment Elevation Myocardial Infarction (FAMOUS NSTEMI) is the first multicenter randomized trial comparing FFR-guided management and angiography-guided standard care, specifically targeting subjects with NSTEMI.[39] In this study, a total of 350 NSTEMI subjects with greater than 1 coronary stenosis greater than 30% of the lumen diameter assessed visually were randomized to FFR-guided management or standard angiography-guided management.[39] The proportion of subjects initially treated with medical therapy was significantly higher in the FFR-guided group (22.7% vs 13.2%, $P = .02$).[39] However, the reduction in major cardiovascular events seen in the subgroup analysis of subjects enrolled in FAME trial[3] was not noted here. There was a trend toward decreased rate of procedure-related myocardial infarction and increased risk of spontaneous myocardial infarction during long-term follow-up in subjects in whom revascularization was deferred based on FFR.[39]

Given the lack of consistency in the limited number of trials conducted among NSTEMI subjects, and the small sample sizes, the prognostic benefit of FFR-guided revascularization in NSTEMI remains controversial until further large-scale multicenter trials are conducted. Currently, it seems that FFR-guided revascularization, especially in the nonculprit vessels in NSTEMI may be helpful in reducing the number of unnecessary interventions without affecting the overall long-term clinical outcomes.

SUMMARY

In conclusion, though the literature is limited, it seems that FFR-guided revascularization may be safely extended to clinical scenarios outside of focal lesions in stable coronary artery disease (tandem, bifurcation, left main lesions, or ACS). The unique changes in fluid hemodynamics that occur in each of these situations should be taken into account when interpreting FFR in these situations. Future large-scale randomized trials are warranted to definitively support the long-term safety of this approach in each of these scenarios.

REFERENCES

1. Pijls NH, van Son JA, Kirkeeide RL, et al. Experimental basis of determining maximum coronary, myocardial, and collateral blood flow by pressure measurements for assessing functional stenosis severity before and after percutaneous transluminal coronary angioplasty. Circulation 1993;87(4):1354–67.

2. Pijls NH, van Schaardenburgh P, Manoharan G, et al. Percutaneous coronary intervention of functionally nonsignificant stenosis: 5-year follow-up of the DEFER Study. J Am Coll Cardiol 2007;49(21):2105–11.

3. Tonino PA, De Bruyne B, Pijls NH, et al. Fractional flow reserve versus angiography for guiding percutaneous coronary intervention. N Engl J Med 2009;360(3):213–24.

4. De Bruyne B, Fearon WF, Pijls NH, et al. Fractional flow reserve-guided PCI for stable coronary artery disease. N Engl J Med 2014;37(13):1208–17.

5. De Bruyne B, Pijls NH, Heyndrickx GR, et al. Pressure-derived fractional flow reserve to assess serial epicardial stenoses: theoretical basis and animal validation. Circulation 2000;101(15):1840–7.

6. Pijls NH, De Bruyne B, Bech GJ, et al. Coronary pressure measurement to assess the hemodynamic significance of serial stenoses within one coronary artery: validation in humans. Circulation 2000;102(19):2371–7.

7. Gould KL, Nakagawa Y, Nakagawa K, et al. Frequency and clinical implications of fluid dynamically significant diffuse coronary artery disease manifest as graded, longitudinal, base-to-apex myocardial perfusion abnormalities by noninvasive positron emission tomography. Circulation 2000;101(16):1931–9.

8. Seiler C, Kirkeeide RL, Gould KL. Basic structure-function relations of the epicardial coronary vascular tree. Basis of quantitative coronary arteriography for diffuse coronary artery disease. Circulation 1992;85(6):1987–2003.

9. Kim HL, Koo BK, Nam CW, et al. Clinical and physiological outcomes of fractional flow reserve-guided percutaneous coronary intervention in patients with serial stenoses within one coronary artery. JACC Cardiovasc Interv 2012;5(10):1013–8.

10. Park SJ, Ahn JM, Pijls NH, et al. Validation of functional state of coronary tandem lesions using computational flow dynamics. Am J Cardiol 2012;110(11):1578–84.

11. Louvard Y, Thomas M, Dzavik V, et al. Classification of coronary artery bifurcation lesions and treatments: time for a consensus! Catheter Cardiovasc Interv 2008;71(2):175–83.

12. Koo BK, De Bruyne B. FFR in bifurcation stenting: what have we learned? EuroIntervention 2010;6(Suppl J):J94–8.

13. Ziaee A, Parham WA, Herrmann SC, et al. Lack of relation between imaging and physiology in ostial coronary artery narrowings. Am J Cardiol 2004;93(11):1404–7. A9.

14. Koo BK, Waseda K, Kang HJ, et al. Anatomic and functional evaluation of bifurcation lesions undergoing percutaneous coronary intervention. Circ Cardiovasc Interv 2010;3(2):113–9.

15. Hildick-Smith D, de Belder AJ, Cooter N, et al. Randomized trial of simple versus complex drug-eluting stenting for bifurcation lesions: the British Bifurcation Coronary Study: old, new, and evolving strategies. Circulation 2010;121(10):1235–43.

16. Niemela M, Kervinen K, Erglis A, et al. Randomized comparison of final kissing balloon dilatation versus

no final kissing balloon dilatation in patients with coronary bifurcation lesions treated with main vessel stenting: the Nordic-Baltic Bifurcation Study III. Circulation 2011;123(1):79–86.

17. Colombo A, Bramucci E, Sacca S, et al. Randomized study of the crush technique versus provisional side-branch stenting in true coronary bifurcations: the CACTUS (Coronary Bifurcations: Application of the Crushing Technique Using Sirolimus-Eluting Stents) Study. Circulation 2009; 119(1):71–8.

18. Williams AR, Koo BK, Gundert TJ, et al. Local hemodynamic changes caused by main branch stent implantation and subsequent virtual side branch balloon angioplasty in a representative coronary bifurcation. J Appl Physiol (1985) 2010;109(2): 532–40.

19. Gao XF, Zhang YJ, Tian NL, et al. Stenting strategy for coronary artery bifurcation with drug-eluting stents: a meta-analysis of nine randomised trials and systematic review. EuroIntervention 2014; 10(5):561–9.

20. Koo BK, Park KW, Kang HJ, et al. Physiological evaluation of the provisional side-branch intervention strategy for bifurcation lesions using fractional flow reserve. Eur Heart J 2008;29(6): 726–32.

21. Lee BK, Choi HH, Hong KS, et al. Efficacy of fractional flow reserve measurements at side branch vessels treated with the crush stenting technique in true coronary bifurcation lesions. Clin Cardiol 2010;33(8):490–4.

22. Park SH, Koo BK. Clinical applications of fractional flow reserve in bifurcation lesions. J Geriatr Cardiol 2012;9(3):278–84.

23. Ratcliffe JA, Huang Y, Kwan T. A novel technique in the use of fractional flow reserve in coronary artery bifurcation lesions. Int J Angiol 2012;21(1): 59–62.

24. Yusuf S, Zucker D, Peduzzi P, et al. Effect of coronary artery bypass graft surgery on survival: overview of 10-year results from randomised trials by the Coronary Artery Bypass Graft Surgery Trialists Collaboration. Lancet 1994;344(8922):563–70.

25. Puri R, Kapadia SR, Nicholls SJ, et al. Optimizing outcomes during left main percutaneous coronary intervention with intravascular ultrasound and fractional flow reserve: the current state of evidence. JACC Cardiovasc Interv 2012;5(7):697–707.

26. Lindstaedt M, Spiecker M, Perings C, et al. How good are experienced interventional cardiologists at predicting the functional significance of intermediate or equivocal left main coronary artery stenoses? Int J Cardiol 2007;120(2):254–61.

27. Hamilos M, Muller O, Cuisset T, et al. Long-term clinical outcome after fractional flow reserve-guided treatment in patients with angiographically

28. Courtis J, Rodes-Cabau J, Larose E, et al. Usefulness of coronary fractional flow reserve measurements in guiding clinical decisions in intermediate or equivocal left main coronary stenoses. Am J Cardiol 2009;103(7):943–9.

29. Bulkley BH, Roberts WC. Atherosclerotic narrowing of the left main coronary artery. A necropsy analysis of 152 patients with fatal coronary heart disease and varying degrees of left main narrowing. Circulation 1976;53(5):823–8.

30. Yong AS, Daniels D, De Bruyne B, et al. Fractional flow reserve assessment of left main stenosis in the presence of downstream coronary stenoses. Circ Cardiovasc Interv 2013;6(2):161–5.

31. Jasti V, Ivan E, Yalamanchili V, et al. Correlations between fractional flow reserve and intravascular ultrasound in patients with an ambiguous left main coronary artery stenosis. Circulation 2004; 110(18):2831–6.

32. Jeremias A, Whitbourn RJ, Filardo SD, et al. Adequacy of intracoronary versus intravenous adenosine-induced maximal coronary hyperemia for fractional flow reserve measurements. Am Heart J 2000;140(4):651–7.

33. Lotfi A, Jeremias A, Fearon WF, et al. Expert consensus statement on the use of fractional flow reserve, intravascular ultrasound, and optical coherence tomography: a consensus statement of the society of cardiovascular angiography and interventions. Catheter Cardiovasc Interv 2014;83(4): 509–18.

34. De Bruyne B, Adjedj J. Fractional flow reserve in acute coronary syndromes. Eur Heart J 2015;36(2): 75–6.

35. Tamita K, Akasaka T, Takagi T, et al. Effects of microvascular dysfunction on myocardial fractional flow reserve after percutaneous coronary intervention in patients with acute myocardial infarction. Catheter Cardiovasc Interv 2002;57(4):452–9.

36. De Bruyne B, Pijls NH, Bartunek J, et al. Fractional flow reserve in patients with prior myocardial infarction. Circulation 2001;104(2):157–62.

37. Leesar MA, Abdul-Baki T, Akkus NI, et al. Use of fractional flow reserve versus stress perfusion scintigraphy after unstable angina. J Am Coll Cardiol 2003;41(7):1115–21.

38. Sels JW, Tonino PA, Siebert U, et al. Fractional flow reserve in unstable angina and non-ST-segment elevation myocardial infarction experience from the FAME (Fractional flow reserve versus Angiography for Multivessel Evaluation) study. JACC Cardiovasc Interv 2011;4(11):1183–9.

39. Layland J, Oldroyd KG, Curzen N, et al. Fractional flow reserve vs angiography in guiding management to optimize outcomes in non-ST-segment

elevation myocardial infarction: the British Heart Foundation FAMOUS-NSTEMI randomized trial. Eur Heart J 2015;36(2):100–11.

40. Samady H, Lepper W, Powers ER, et al. Fractional flow reserve of infarct-related arteries identifies reversible defects on noninvasive myocardial perfusion imaging early after myocardial infarction. J Am Coll Cardiol 2006;47(11):2187–93.

41. Lekston A, Tajstra M, Gasior M, et al. Impact of multivessel coronary disease on one-year clinical outcomes and five-year mortality in patients with ST-elevation myocardial infarction undergoing percutaneous coronary intervention. Kardiol Pol 2011;69(4):336–43.

42. O'Gara PT, Kushner FG, Ascheim DD, et al. 2013 ACCF/AHA guideline for the management of ST-elevation myocardial infarction: a report of the American College of Cardiology Foundation/ American Heart Association Task Force on Practice Guidelines. Catheter Cardiovasc Interv 2013;82(1): E1–27.

43. Rosner GF, Kirtane AJ, Genereux P, et al. Impact of the presence and extent of incomplete angiographic revascularization after percutaneous coronary intervention in acute coronary syndromes: the Acute Catheterization and Urgent Intervention Triage Strategy (ACUITY) trial. Circulation 2012; 125(21):2613–20.

44. Wald DS, Morris JK, Wald NJ, et al. Randomized trial of preventive angioplasty in myocardial infarction. N Engl J Med 2013;369(12):1115–23.

45. Ntalianis A, Sels JW, Davidavicius G, et al. Fractional flow reserve for the assessment of nonculprit coronary artery stenoses in patients with acute myocardial infarction. JACC Cardiovasc Interv 2010;3(12):1274–81.

Noninvasive Fractional Flow Reserve Derived from Coronary Computed Tomography Angiography for the Diagnosis of Lesion-specific Ischemia

Ibrahim Danad, MD, Lohendran Baskaran, MD,
James K. Min, MD*

KEYWORDS

- Fractional flow reserve • Coronary CT angiography • FFR$_{CT}$ • Coronary artery disease

---

KEY POINTS

- Fractional flow reserve derived from coronary computed tomography angiography (FFR$_{CT}$) has emerged as a powerful tool for the assessment of flow-limiting coronary stenoses.
- To date, FFR$_{CT}$ is the only noninvasive imaging modality for the depiction of lesion-specific ischemia and large prospective multicenter studies have established its high diagnostic value.
- The nature of FFR$_{CT}$ allows the prediction of functional outcome of coronary stenting, which will expand the role of cardiac CT in the evaluation and management of coronary artery disease.

INTRODUCTION

Coronary computed tomography angiography (CCTA) is a noninvasive alternative for the evaluation of coronary anatomy. An array of studies have established its high sensitivity and negative predictive value (NPV),[1,2] rendering it an excellent tool for the rule out of obstructive coronary artery disease. Yet, CCTA tends to overestimate the degree of stenosis when compared with invasive coronary angiography (ICA),[2] which may prompt more downstream testing and unnecessary referrals to the catheterization laboratory.[3] In addition, CCTA is a purely anatomic imaging modality unable to determine the physiologic severity of coronary lesions, and even amongst CCTA-identified significant lesions confirmed by ICA, approximately half of them are found to be flow-limiting.[4,5] Therefore, functional testing of coronary stenoses deemed significant by CCTA is mandatory, not only to improve diagnostic accuracy, but also to enhance clinical decision-making on the need for a coronary revascularization. Fractional flow reserve (FFR) is considered the gold standard for determining the functional repercussion of angiographically intermediate stenosis.[6,7] It has been demonstrated that FFR-based guidance of coronary revascularization relieves symptoms and improves outcomes.[8–10] However, the

---

Research funding: This article was funded, in part, by grants from the National Heart, Lung, and Blood Institute (R01 HL111141, R01 HL115150 and R01 HL118019), as well as from a generous gift from the Dalio Foundation.
Disclosures: J.K. Min serves as a consultant to GE Healthcare, HeartFlow, Abbott Vascular, and Philips Healthcare.
Department of Radiology, Dalio Institute of Cardiovascular Imaging, New York-Presbyterian Hospital, Weill Cornell Medical College, 413 East 69th Street, New York, NY 10021, USA
* Corresponding author. Dalio Institute of Cardiovascular Imaging, New York-Presbyterian Hospital, Weill Cornell Medical College, 413 East 69th Street, Suite 108, New York, NY 10021.
E-mail address: jkm2001@med.cornell.edu

invasive nature of FFR limits its application to broad populations as an initial diagnostic test. For the noninvasive diagnosis and management of coronary artery disease (CAD), detection of myocardial ischemia is indicated, and nuclear imaging modalities, such as single-photon emission computed tomography (SPECT) and PET have traditionally been assigned to this task. Importantly, detection of myocardial perfusion with these techniques comes at a cost of patient inconvenience and radiation exposure. Recently, a novel method has been described that applies computational fluid dynamics to derive FFR from traditional CCTA images (FFR$_{CT}$), obviating the need of additional imaging, modifications of computed tomography (CT) acquisition protocols, or administration of medications.[11] Notably, prospective multicenter studies demonstrated FFR$_{CT}$ to exhibit high diagnostic accuracy for identification of flow-limiting CAD.[11–13] As such, FFR$_{CT}$ may become a method that provides complementary information on coronary anatomy and the physiologic implications of coronary stenoses in patients evaluated for CAD.

FRACTIONAL FLOW RESERVE FOR THE ASSESSMENT OF LESION-SPECIFIC ISCHEMIA

FFR measurements in the presence of coronary stenoses have proved to yield useful information on the functional severity of coronary lesions.[14] FFR is an index and is defined as the ratio of hyperemic maximum coronary flow in a stenotic artery to maximum coronary flow in the same artery if it was hypothetically completely normal.

The ratio of the 2 flows is expressed as the ratio of 2 pressures, namely the pressure proximal and distal to the stenosis (Fig. 1). The relationship between coronary flow and FFR was investigated in the early 1990s by Pijls and colleagues[15] in animal models, providing the basis for the concept of pressure measurements as a derivative of coronary flow and subsequent pathophysiologic severity of coronary artery stenoses. As such, normal myocardial blood flow is considered a prerequisite for the absence of hyperemic intracoronary pressure gradients.[15] Interestingly, the clinical feasibility of FFR was shown in 22 patients with an isolated stenosis in the left anterior descending artery, whereby FFR was compared against a background of quantitative [^{15}O]H$_2$O PET.[16] De Bruyne and colleagues[16] demonstrated that FFR was closely related to the relative flow reserve obtained by [^{15}O]H$_2$O PET ($r = 0.86$); however, coronary pressure and myocardial blood flow are not interchangeable and discrepancies between these 2 parameters do not imply the failure of either technique, but merely reflect the heterogeneous nature of coronary atherosclerosis spanning the gamut from focal obstructive CAD to coronary microvascular dysfunction.[17–19] However, to date, FFR is the only technique for the detection of ischemia that has been prospectively validated against multiple reference standards,[14] using the so-called Bayesian approach, rendering it a robust and reliable tool. The importance of FFR measurements for the evaluation of CAD has been demonstrated by the landmark FAME (Fractional Flow Reserve vs Angiography for Multivessel Evaluation) trial, which showed that FFR-guided stenting improved patient outcome

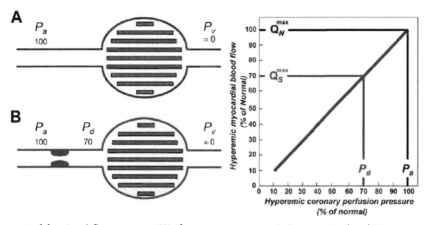

Fig. 1. Concept of fractional flow reserve. (A) If no coronary stenosis is present, the driving pressure reflects maximum coronary flow (100%). In the presence of a given epicardial stenosis (B), driving pressure in this example is no longer 100%, but only 70%. As such, myocardial blood flow is only 70% of maximum and FFR (Pd/Pa) = 0.70. *From* Pijls NH, Tanaka N, Fearon WF. Functional assessment of coronary stenoses: can we live without it? Eur Heart J 2013;34(18):1335–44; with permission.

as compared with percutaneous coronary intervention (PCI) guided by angiography alone.[20] Notably, the results of the FAME trial suggest that stenting of non–hemodynamically significant lesions (FFR >0.80) is potentially detrimental.[20] Apparently, the number of events associated with a stent implantation outweighs the rate of events caused by a non–functionally relevant lesion that is treated by optimal medical therapy alone. Furthermore, the FAME-2 trial demonstrated that FFR-guided revascularization reduced urgent revascularizations substantially in those patients with a functionally relevant lesion (FFR ≤0.80) compared with optimal medical therapy.[10] FFR has been clinically embraced as the functional gold standard and current guidelines advocate its use as a tool to guide clinical decision-making with regard to the assessment of functional severity of stenosis and subsequent revascularizations.[6,7]

NONINVASIVE FRACTIONAL FLOW RESERVE COMPUTED FROM STANDARD CORONARY COMPUTED TOMOGRAPHY ANGIOGRAPHY IMAGES

The scientific principles and the method of calculating FFR from standard CCTA images by computational fluid dynamics has been described by Taylor and colleagues[21] in great detail. Noninvasive computational FFR from standard coronary CT images requires an anatomic model of the coronary arteries, a physiologic model of coronary and systemic circulation, and a numerical solution of the laws of physics governing fluid dynamics (Fig. 2). First,

the required 3-dimensional anatomical model consisting of the aortic root and the coronary tree is directly extracted from the CCTA data. The physiologic models pertain to 3 principles with regard to baseline coronary flow, coronary microvascular resistance at rest, and to the vasodilator response of the microcirculation to adenosine. Baseline coronary flow is calculated as a derivative of myocardial mass. Choy and Kassab[22] showed that a linear relationship exists between coronary artery flow and myocardial mass. As such, baseline coronary flow can be quantified relative to the myocardial volume, which is a surrogate for mass, as assessed by CT. The second principle states that coronary microvascular resistance during resting conditions is inversely related to the diameter of the vessel pertaining to the flow-pressure relationship, as described by Poiseuille's law. Third, because FFR$_{CT}$ is derived from standard CCTA without any modifications to the acquisition protocol, stressor agents are not used to calculate FFR$_{CT}$. In lieu of adenosine, a simulation model is used to determine the decrease in coronary microvascular resistance if adenosine was administered at a rate of 140 µg · kg^{-1} · min^{-1}, which is the recommended dose for FFR measurements.[14] As such, this assumptive model allows computational modeling of FFR during hyperemia. Nevertheless, this assumption on alterations in resistance as a result of adenosine are based on the work of Wilson and colleagues,[23] who showed hyperemic coronary resistance fell to 0.24 of the resting value with the intravenous administration of 140 µg · kg^{-1} · min^{-1} adenosine, which enabled near-maximal vasodilation

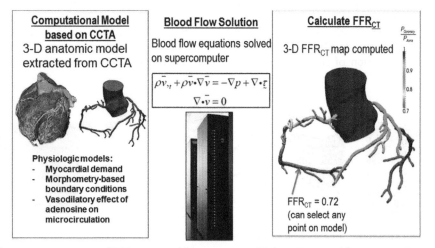

Fig. 2. Schematic presentation of FFR computed from coronary CT data. Fractional flow reserve (FFR$_{CT}$) can now be accurately computed from a typically acquired coronary CT angiography, without the need for additional imaging, additional medications or modification of image acquisition protocols.

equivalent to the dilation elicited by intracoronary papaverine. Altogether, the integration of these physiologic models to the patient-specific anatomy of the aortic root and coronary tree allow for the calculation of a computational fluid dynamics–based FFR value (see Fig. 2).

EVIDENCE IN THE LITERATURE ON THE DIAGNOSTIC VALUE OF FFR_CT

FFR_CT has emerged as a novel technique for the noninvasive depiction of lesion-specific ischemia (Fig. 3), with mounting evidence reporting its high diagnostic performance for the detection of hemodynamic significant CAD. Interestingly, although the absolute number of studies on FFR_CT is small when compared with traditional imaging modalities, such as SPECT, the prospective multicenter design of the FFR_CT studies renders their obtained results robust and highly generalizable. Furthermore, due to its ability to detect lesion-specific ischemia, the use of FFR as a reference standard is unquestioned, which is in contrast to nuclear imaging and MRI perfusion studies that have almost exclusively been refereed against an ICA comparator.

The diagnostic performance of FFR_CT was first reported in the prospective multicenter DISCOVER-FLOW (Diagnosis of Ischemia-Causing Coronary Stenoses by Noninvasive Fractional Flow Reserve Computed From Coronary Computed Tomographic Angiograms) trial, in which FFR_CT was performed in 103 (159 vessels) patients with suspected or known CAD who underwent both CCTA and ICA in conjunction with FFR measurements.[11] Koo and colleagues[11] found a per-vessel accuracy, sensitivity, specificity, positive predictive value (PPV), and NPV for FFR_CT of 84.3%, 87.9%, 82.2%, 73.9%, and 92.2%, respectively, and 58.5%, 91.4%, 39.6%, 46.5%, and 88.9% for CCTA for the detection of significant coronary stenoses as indicated by FFR. Similar to per-vessel analysis, a higher accuracy was obtained by FFR_CT on a per-patient basis. Application of FFR_CT to CCTA augments the diagnostic accuracy of CCTA by reducing the rate of false-positive lesions incorrectly classified by anatomic stenosis severity alone. Notably, the ability of FFR_CT to detect flow-limiting CAD was significantly improved, with an increase in the area under the curve (AUC) as compared with CCTA of 0.90 versus 0.75, respectively (P<.001).[11]

The second study investigating the clinical value of FFR_CT was the DeFACTO (Determination of Fractional Flow Reserve by Anatomic Computed Tomographic Angiography) trial, which was a prospective multicenter study involving 252 patients with suspected or known CAD from 17 centers in 5 countries.[12] A total of 252 patients were included and, similar to the DISCOVER-FLOW trial, FFR_CT was superior to CCTA with regard to discrimination of lesion-specific ischemia.[12] Sensitivity, specificity, PPV, NPV, and accuracy were 84%, 42%, 61%, 72%, and 64% for CCTA alone and 90%, 54%, 67%, 84%, and 73% on a per-patient analysis for the combined assessment consisting of FFR_CT and CCTA. Importantly, although FFR_CT improved diagnostic accuracy of CCTA as reflected by significantly higher AUC of 0.81 versus 0.68 for CCTA alone (P<.001), the study failed to achieve the prespecified diagnostic endpoint of an accuracy of at least 70% as determined by the lower bound of the 95% confidence interval, being only 68% for FFR_CT.[12] Notably, the sensitivity and NPV of CCTA were only 84% and 72%, which is in marked contrast with CCTA's unambiguously high sensitivity and NPV greater than 90% as reported in the literature. This may be attributable to the quality of the CT acquisition, which may hamper interpretation and grading of stenosis severity. Based on the DeFACTO data, Leipsic and colleagues[24]

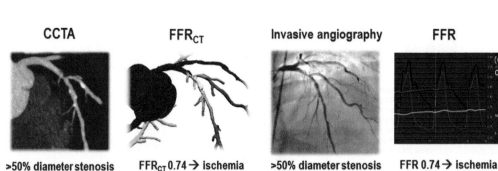

CCTA   **FFR_CT**   **Invasive angiography**   **FFR**

>50% diameter stenosis   FFR_CT 0.74 → ischemia   >50% diameter stenosis   FFR 0.74 → ischemia

Fig. 3. Noninvasive detection of lesion-specific ischemia by FFR_CT. A case example of epicardial lesion deemed significant on CCTA and ICA (both >50%), which is shown by FFR_CT to be indeed hemodynamically significant (FFR_CT = 0.74) and confirmed by invasive FFR (0.74).

showed that the use of beta-blockers and nitroglycerin might improve the diagnostic performance of FFR$_{CT}$. Sensitivity remained unchanged irrespective of beta-blocker and nitroglycerine use, whereas specificity was 66.4% in patients who received beta-blockers and nitroglycerin compared with 51.4% (P = .03) in medication-naïve patients.[24] These findings argue in favor of an image-quality–dependent improvement of FFR$_{CT}$. However, these results were based on a post hoc analysis based on the DeFACTO trial and should be interpreted cautiously. Another study showed that FFR$_{CT}$ is impervious to factors known to adversely affect CCTA image quality, such as heart rate, signal-to-noise-ratio, coronary calcifications, motion or misalignment artifacts, and poor contrast enhancement.[25] Nevertheless, the current CT guidelines advocate for administration of beta-blockers and nitroglycerin to improve image quality of cardiac CT, and the results of Leipsic and colleagues[24,26] show the importance of adherence to practice guidelines for image acquisition to optimize performance of both CCTA and FFR$_{CT}$.

Therefore, in contrast to the previous studies, the most recent large study on FFR$_{CT}$, the NXT trial (Analysis of Coronary Blood Flow Using CT Angiography: Next Steps), applied stringent criteria with regard to CT acquisition, particularly focusing on heart-rate control and administration of prescan nitroglycerine, and used the latest generation of FFR$_{CT}$ computational algorithms and the most recent software for automated image processing.[13] As such, there was a good correlation between FFR$_{CT}$ and FFR (r = 0.82, P<.001). In the NXT trial, among 254 subjects, detection of hemodynamically significant CAD by CCTA yielded a sensitivity, specificity, PPV, NPV, and accuracy of 94%, 34%, 40%, 92%, and 53%, respectively, and 86%, 79%, 65%, 93%, and 81% for FFR$_{CT}$. The diagnostic performance of FFR$_{CT}$ was significantly higher compared with CCTA as reflected by an AUC of 0.90 versus 0.81 (P<.01), respectively, which was mainly driven by a correct reclassification of CCTA false-positive findings.[13] Norgaard and colleagues[13] showed that FFR$_{CT}$ was able to reclassify a remarkable number of patients (68%) with a false-positive CCTA scan as true negatives. **Fig. 4** shows a clinical example wherein FFR$_{CT}$ correctly reclassified a false-positive CCTA scan. Of note, strict adherence to the best practices for CT image acquisition resulted in a high NPV of 93%,[13] which is in line with the large body of literature establishing CCTA's role for the rule out of obstructive CAD.[1] Notably, more than 90% of patients in the NXT trial had an epicardial lesion of intermediate angiographic severity (30%–70%), a diagnostically challenging population where FFR is considered to be of particular benefit to guide clinical decision-making. Consequently, Nakazato and colleagues[27] showed that, among 82 patients of the DeFACTO trial who were diagnosed with intermediate coronary stenoses on ICA ranging between 30% and 69%, FFR$_{CT}$ continued to possess an incremental diagnostic value over CCTA as reflected by a significantly higher AUC for FFR$_{CT}$ of 0.81 compared with 0.50 for CT alone (P<.01).

The prospective multicenter design of the aforementioned studies renders their results highly generalizable. Indeed, a recently published post hoc analysis performed in the Japanese population of the NXT trial revealed similar diagnostic performance of FFR$_{CT}$ among 47 subjects with coronary artery calcium (CAC) scores less than 1000 as compared with the initial results of the NXT trial with sensitivity, specificity, PPV, NPV, and accuracy being 100%, 75.8%, 63.6%, 100%, and 83.0%, respectively.[28] In spite of this, however, the observations by Miyoshi and colleagues[28] also pointed out that severe calcifications may hamper the ability of FFR$_{CT}$ to accurately delineate the functional relevance of a given epicardial lesion. Accordingly, if subjects with heavy calcifications

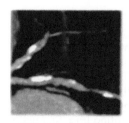 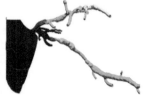 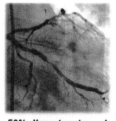 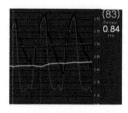

>50% diameter stenosis   **FFR$_{CT}$ 0.85 → no ischemia**   **>50% diameter stenosis**   **FFR 0.84 → no ischemia**

Fig. 4. FFR$_{CT}$ reduces the number of false-positive CT findings. A case example of a calcified plaque that appears obstructive on CCTA and ICA (both >50%), but FFR$_{CT}$ (0.85) shows no impediment of coronary flow, which is confirmed by invasive FFR (0.84).

(Agatston score >1000) were included in the analysis, sensitivity, specificity, PPV, NPV, and accuracy for FFR$_{CT}$ (CCTA) were 100% (100%), 63.4% (26.8%), 51.6% (34.8%), 100% (100%), and 74.0% (47.0%), which is remarkably lower than the results obtained by Norgaard and colleagues,[13] albeit obtained in a small sample of patients (n = 57). Yet, FFR$_{CT}$ continued to exhibit a higher accuracy than CCTA and appears to be less influenced by factors such as heavy calcifications, known for adversely affecting CT image quality.[28]

Interestingly, discordances between invasive FFR and FFR$_{CT}$ do not necessarily arise from the failure of FFR$_{CT}$ to depict hemodynamically significant CAD, but may be attributable to the methodology used. For example, in clinical practice, only arteries with a suitable diameter for coronary revascularizations are interrogated by FFR, whereas distally located stenoses are often neglected. Unlike invasive FFR, CT-derived FFR values can be computed for all vessels. Hence, inherent to its ease of application, an important bias is posed, because the present use of FFR$_{CT}$ appears to be different from invasive FFR. As such, to ensure a fair comparison with invasive FFR in terms of both diagnostic accuracy and clinical decision-making, the implementation of FFR$_{CT}$ needs to be in adherence to the clinical rules applied for FFR. In this regard, one study by Thompson and colleagues[29] evaluated the diagnostic performance of FFR$_{CT}$ when subjected to the same clinical rules as invasive FFR so as to reflect true clinical practice with regard to FFR measurements. As a consequence, stenoses less than 30% diameter were assigned an FFR$_{CT}$ value of 0.90, subtotal stenoses (>90%) were assumed to be functionally significant and were assigned an FFR$_{CT}$ value of 0.50, whereas vessels with a diameter <2 mm were excluded from FFR$_{CT}$ measurements. With this approach, Thompson and colleagues[29] reported a per-patient sensitivity, specificity, PPV, NPV, and accuracy among 252 patients of 86%, 82%, 61%, 95%, and 83%, respectively, for FFR$_{CT}$ to discriminate lesion-specific ischemia. Of interest, when evaluated in accordance with its expected use, accuracy of FFR$_{CT}$ improved significantly from 72% to 83% (P<.01), which was primarily driven by an increase in specificity from 54% to 82% (P<.001). Additionally, it has been shown that the diagnostic performance of FFR$_{CT}$ remained high, irrespective of age and gender.[29] The robustness of this technique also is reflected by its high reproducibility with repeated measurements with a coefficient of variation of 3.4%, equal to the within-patient variation of 3.3% for invasive FFR measurements.[30]

COST-EFFECTIVENESS OF FFR$_{CT}$

Although it has been shown that FFR$_{CT}$ improves diagnostic accuracy of CCTA through a reduction in the number of false-positive scans, the cost-effectiveness of this tool has yet to be established in real patient data. However, one might envision FFR$_{CT}$ to reduce overall CAD-related spending due to a more judicious referral of patients to the catheterization laboratory. In this regard, 2 studies have recently evaluated the cost-effectiveness of FFR$_{CT}$ in 2 different populations using a cost-effectiveness simulation analysis.[31,32] The first study was by Hlatky and colleagues[31] amongst 96 patients who were included in the DISCOVER-flow trial. They found that a strategy of initial CCTA with FFR$_{CT}$ for patients with 50% or more stenosis and referral of only those patients with an FFR$_{CT}$ of 0.80 or less to the catheterization laboratory and subsequent PCI will reduce the number of invasive coronary angiographies by 51% as compared with a strategy whereby patients underwent ICA as an initial diagnostic test.[31] In addition, the use of FFR$_{CT}$ as gatekeeper for ICA and PCI was demonstrated to be the most cost-effective approach. Similarly, based on the NXT trial database, Kimura and colleagues[32] reported a 30% reduction in costs and importantly a 61% reduction in the number of referrals to ICA when using FFR$_{CT}$ as gatekeeper to the catheterization laboratory. However, both studies used simulation models to determine overall costs, and the cost-effectiveness of FFR$_{CT}$ in real patient data is not established yet. It is anticipated, however, that the ongoing PLATFORM (Prospective LongitudinAl Trial of FFR$_{CT}$: Outcome and Resource Impacts; NCT01943903) trial will provide important evidence with regard to outcome and cost-effectiveness of an FFR$_{CT}$-guided evaluation as compared with standard care of practice.

FUTURE PERSPECTIVES

Given the unique feature of FFR$_{CT}$ being derived from standard CCTA images without any modifications to CT acquisition protocols, the same computational fluid dynamics models may also enable the prediction of functional outcome by coronary stenting (Fig. 5). Enlargement of the affected lumen according to the diameter of the proximal and distal segments, to virtually eliminate an epicardial stenosis, allows for the assessment of an FFR value after

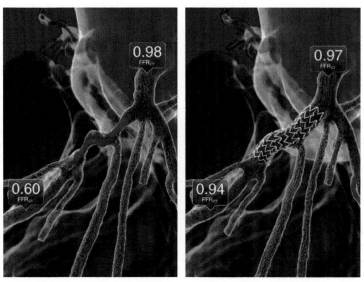

Fig. 5. Virtual stenting by FFR$_{CT}$ to predict functional outcome of coronary stenting.

successful revascularization. This is of importance, because abnormal pressure gradients after stenting are a strong predictor of adverse outcome.[33] Kim and colleagues[34] demonstrated the clinical feasibility of virtual stenting by FFR$_{CT}$ to predict functional outcomes after a coronary PCI. In this study, consisting of 44 patients with 48 arteries containing hemodynamically significant coronary lesions, a statistically significant correlation between computed FFR$_{CT}$ after virtual stenting and invasively measured FFR after PCI ($r = 0.55$, $P<.001$) was found.[34] The average FFR pre-PCI was 0.70 ± 0.14 and increased to 0.90 ± 0.05 after coronary stenting, whereas FFR$_{CT}$ showed a concomitant increase from 0.70 ± 0.15 to

0.88 ± 0.05, respectively. The diagnostic performance of FFR$_{CT}$ to predict residual ischemia was excellent, as reflected by a sensitivity, specificity, PPV, NPV, and accuracy of 100%, 96%, 50%, 100%, and 96%, respectively.[34] The study by Kim and colleagues[34] is the first to demonstrate the feasibility of virtual stenting and the results are promising, albeit in a small patient cohort. The ability of FFR$_{CT}$ to predict functional outcome after coronary stenting is exemplified in **Fig. 6**. Nevertheless, the implementation of virtual stenting will broaden the horizons of cardiac CT and has opened new doors for planning optimal treatment strategies and has brought patient-specific and vessel-specific treatment of CAD within reach.

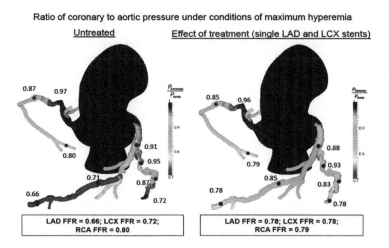

Fig. 6. Feasibility of virtual stenting by FFR$_{CT}$ to predict functional outcome of coronary revascularizations. A flow-limiting stenosis in the left anterior descending (LAD) and left circumflex artery with concomitant FFR values of 0.66, and 0.72, respectively (left figure). The predicted effect of a revascularization will result in an increase of FFR from 0.66 to 0.78 in the LAD artery, whereas FFR will improve from 0.72 to 0.78 in the LCX artery (right figure). RCA, right coronary artery.

SUMMARY

FFR$_{CT}$ has emerged as a powerful tool for the assessment of flow-limiting coronary stenoses. To date, FFR$_{CT}$ is the only noninvasive imaging modality for the depiction of lesion-specific ischemia, and large prospective multicenter studies have established its high diagnostic value. The nature of FFR$_{CT}$ allows the prediction of functional outcome of coronary stenting, which will expand the role of cardiac CT in the evaluation and management of CAD.

REFERENCES

1. Sun Z, Lin C, Davidson R, et al. Diagnostic value of 64-slice CT angiography in coronary artery disease: a systematic review. Eur J Radiol 2008;67:78–84.

2. Budoff MJ, Dowe D, Jollis JG, et al. Diagnostic performance of 64-multidetector row coronary computed tomographic angiography for evaluation of coronary artery stenosis in individuals without known coronary artery disease: results from the prospective multicenter ACCURACY (Assessment by Coronary Computed Tomographic Angiography of Individuals Undergoing Invasive Coronary Angiography) trial. J Am Coll Cardiol 2008;52:1724–32.

3. Shreibati JB, Baker LC, Hlatky MA. Association of coronary CT angiography or stress testing with subsequent utilization and spending among Medicare beneficiaries. JAMA 2011;306:2128–36.

4. Gaemperli O, Schepis T, Valenta I, et al. Functionally relevant coronary artery disease: comparison of 64-section CT angiography with myocardial perfusion SPECT. Radiology 2008;248:414–23.

5. Danad I, Raijmakers PG, Harms HJ, et al. Effect of cardiac hybrid (1)(5)O-water PET/CT imaging on downstream referral for invasive coronary angiography and revascularization rate. Eur Heart J Cardiovasc Imaging 2014;15:170–9.

6. Task Force on Myocardial Revascularization of the European Society of Cardiology and the European Association for Cardio-Thoracic Surgery, Windecker S, Kolh P, et al. 2014 ESC/EACTS Guidelines on myocardial revascularization: the Task Force on Myocardial Revascularization of the European Society of Cardiology (ESC) and the European Association for Cardio-Thoracic Surgery (EACTS) developed with the special contribution of the European Association of Percutaneous Cardiovascular Interventions (EAPCI). Eur Heart J 2014;35:2541–619.

7. Fihn SD, Blankenship JC, Alexander KP, et al. 2014 ACC/AHA/AATS/PCNA/SCAI/STS focused update of the guideline for the diagnosis and management of patients with stable ischemic heart disease: a report of the American College of Cardiology/ American Heart Association Task Force on Practice Guidelines, and the American Association for Thoracic Surgery, Preventive Cardiovascular Nurses Association, Society for Cardiovascular Angiography and Interventions, and Society of Thoracic Surgeons. J Am Coll Cardiol 2014;64:1929–49.

8. De Bruyne B, Fearon WF, Pijls NH, et al. Fractional flow reserve-guided PCI for stable coronary artery disease. N Engl J Med 2014;371:1208–17.

9. De Bruyne B, Pijls NH, Kalesan B, et al. Fractional flow reserve-guided PCI versus medical therapy in stable coronary disease. N Engl J Med 2012;367: 991–1001.

10. Pijls NH, Fearon WF, Tonino PA, et al. Fractional flow reserve versus angiography for guiding percutaneous coronary intervention in patients with multivessel coronary artery disease: 2-year follow-up of the FAME (Fractional Flow Reserve Versus Angiography for Multivessel Evaluation) study. J Am Coll Cardiol 2010;56:177–84.

11. Koo BK, Erglis A, Doh JH, et al. Diagnosis of ischemia-causing coronary stenoses by noninvasive fractional flow reserve computed from coronary computed tomographic angiograms. Results from the prospective multicenter DISCOVER-FLOW (Diagnosis of Ischemia-Causing Stenoses Obtained Via Noninvasive Fractional Flow Reserve) study. J Am Coll Cardiol 2011;58:1989–97.

12. Min JK, Leipsic J, Pencina MJ, et al. Diagnostic accuracy of fractional flow reserve from anatomic CT angiography. JAMA 2012;308:1237–45.

13. Norgaard BL, Leipsic J, Gaur S, et al. Diagnostic performance of noninvasive fractional flow reserve derived from coronary computed tomography angiography in suspected coronary artery disease: the NXT trial (Analysis of Coronary Blood Flow Using CT Angiography: Next Steps). J Am Coll Cardiol 2014;63:1145–55.

14. Pijls NH, De Bruyne B, Peels K, et al. Measurement of fractional flow reserve to assess the functional severity of coronary-artery stenoses. N Engl J Med 1996;334:1703–8.

15. Pijls NH, van Son JA, Kirkeeide RL, et al. Experimental basis of determining maximum coronary, myocardial, and collateral blood flow by pressure measurements for assessing functional stenosis severity before and after percutaneous transluminal coronary angioplasty. Circulation 1993;87: 1354–67.

16. De Bruyne B, Baudhuin T, Melin JA, et al. Coronary flow reserve calculated from pressure measurements in humans. Validation with positron emission tomography. Circulation 1994;89:1013–22.

17. Johnson NP, Kirkeeide RL, Gould KL. Is discordance of coronary flow reserve and fractional flow reserve due to methodology or clinically relevant

coronary pathophysiology? JACC Cardiovasc Imaging 2012;5:193–202.

18. Schindler TH, Schelbert HR, Quercioli A, et al. Cardiac PET imaging for the detection and monitoring of coronary artery disease and microvascular health. JACC Cardiovasc Imaging 2010;3:623–40.

19. Danad I, Uusitalo V, Kero T, et al. Quantitative assessment of myocardial perfusion in the detection of significant coronary artery disease: cutoff values and diagnostic accuracy of quantitative [(15)O]H2O PET imaging. J Am Coll Cardiol 2014; 64:1464–75.

20. Tonino PA, De Bruyne B, Pijls NH, et al. Fractional flow reserve versus angiography for guiding percutaneous coronary intervention. N Engl J Med 2009; 360:213–24.

21. Taylor CA, Fonte TA, Min JK. Computational fluid dynamics applied to cardiac computed tomography for noninvasive quantification of fractional flow reserve: scientific basis. J Am Coll Cardiol 2013;61:2233–41.

22. Choy JS, Kassab GS. Scaling of myocardial mass to flow and morphometry of coronary arteries. J Appl Physiol 2008;104:1281–6.

23. Wilson RF, Wyche K, Christensen BV, et al. Effects of adenosine on human coronary arterial circulation. Circulation 1990;82:1595–606.

24. Leipsic J, Yang TH, Thompson A, et al. CT angiography (CTA) and diagnostic performance of noninvasive fractional flow reserve: results from the Determination of Fractional Flow Reserve by Anatomic CTA (DeFACTO) study. AJR Am J Roentgenol 2014;202:989–94.

25. Min JK, Koo BK, Erglis A, et al. Effect of image quality on diagnostic accuracy of noninvasive fractional flow reserve: results from the prospective multicenter international DISCOVER-FLOW study. J Cardiovasc Comput Tomogr 2012;6:191–9.

26. Leipsic J, Abbara S, Achenbach S, et al. SCCT guidelines for the interpretation and reporting of coronary CT angiography: a report of the Society of Cardiovascular Computed Tomography Guidelines Committee. J Cardiovasc Comput Tomogr 2014;8:342–58.

27. Nakazato R, Park HB, Berman DS, et al. Noninvasive fractional flow reserve derived from computed tomography angiography for coronary lesions of intermediate stenosis severity: results from the DeFACTO study. Circ Cardiovasc Imaging 2013;6: 881–9.

28. Miyoshi T, Osawa K, Ito H, et al. Non-invasive computed fractional flow reserve from computed tomography (CT) for diagnosing coronary artery disease. Circ J 2015;79:406–12.

29. Thompson AG, Raju R, Blanke P, et al. Diagnostic accuracy and discrimination of ischemia by fractional flow reserve CT using a clinical use rule: results from the determination of fractional flow reserve by anatomic computed tomographic angiography study. J Cardiovasc Comput Tomogr 2015;9:120–8.

30. Gaur S, Bezerra HG, Lassen JF, et al. Fractional flow reserve derived from coronary CT angiography: variation of repeated analyses. J Cardiovasc Comput Tomogr 2014;8:307–14.

31. Hlatky MA, Saxena A, Koo BK, et al. Projected costs and consequences of computed tomography-determined fractional flow reserve. Clin Cardiol 2013;36:743–8.

32. Kimura T, Shiomi H, Kuribayashi S, et al. Cost analysis of non-invasive fractional flow reserve derived from coronary computed tomographic angiography in Japan. Cardiovasc Interv Ther 2015;30: 38–44.

33. Pijls NH, Klauss V, Siebert U, et al. Coronary pressure measurement after stenting predicts adverse events at follow-up: a multicenter registry. Circulation 2002;105:2950–4.

34. Kim KH, Doh JH, Koo BK, et al. A novel noninvasive technology for treatment planning using virtual coronary stenting and computed tomography-derived computed fractional flow reserve. JACC Cardiovasc Interv 2014;7:72–8.

Association of Wall Shear Stress with Coronary Plaque Progression and Transformation

Olivia Y. Hung, MD, PhD[a], Adam J. Brown, MD[b],
Sung Gyun Ahn, MD, PhD[a,c], Alessandro Veneziani, PhD[d],
Don P. Giddens, PhD[e], Habib Samady, MD[f,*]

KEYWORDS

- Wall shear stress • Atherosclerosis • Coronary plaque • Coronary plaque rupture • Intravascular imaging

KEY POINTS

- Wall shear stress (WSS) is the parallel frictional force component that blood exerts on the arterial wall surface as it flows past.
- Computational fluid dynamic simulations are created by fusing intravascular imaging cross-sections and biplane angiography, creating the geometry and using in vivo blood velocity measurements as boundary conditions.
- Sustained abnormal pathologic WSS leads to a proatherogenic endothelial cell phenotype, focal development of atherosclerosis, and adaptive vascular remodeling.
- Rupture occurs when the structural stress within the plaque exceeds material strength; alterations in WSS may be a mechanism in the creation of plaques that are vulnerable to failure.
- Human studies confirm that low WSS is an essential factor in determining focal plaque progression.

INTRODUCTION

In patients with coronary artery disease, plaque progression is a local phenomenon that occurs within an environment of systemic risk factors. It has been observed that atherosclerosis develops preferentially in branching locations and along the inner wall of curvatures,[1] which is consistent with areas of low wall shear stress

Conflicts of Interest: O.Y. Hung is funded by the NIH Ruth L. Kirschstein National Research Service Awards training grant (5T32HL007745) and also has research project support from Gilead Sciences, Medtronic, Volcano Corp and St. Jude Medical. A.J. Brown is funded by the British Heart Foundation (FS/13/33/30168). D.P. Giddens is supported by the Georgia Research Alliance. H. Samady has research project support from Gilead Sciences, Medtronic, Volcano Corp, St. Jude Medical, Toshiba Corp and Abbott Vascular. S.G. Ahn and A. Veneziani have no disclosures to report.
a Division of Cardiology, Department of Medicine, Emory University School of Medicine, 1364 Clifton Road NE, Atlanta, GA 30322, USA; b Department of Cardiovascular Medicine, University of Cambridge, ACCI Level 6, Addenbrooke's Hospital, Hills Road, Cambridge CB2 0QQ, UK; c Division of Cardiology, Yonsei University, Wonju College of Medicine, 20 Ilsan-ro, Wonju 220-701, South Korea; d Department of Mathematics and Computer Science, Emory University, 400 Dowman Drive, Atlanta, GA 30322, USA; e Department of Biomedical Engineering, Georgia Institute of Technology and Emory University, 313 Ferst Dr, Atlanta, GA 30332, USA; f Interventional Cardiology, Division of Cardiology, Department of Medicine, Emory University School of Medicine, 1364 Clifton Road, Suite F606, Atlanta, GA 30322, USA
* Corresponding author.
E-mail address: hsamady@emory.edu

Intervent Cardiol Clin 4 (2015) 491–502
http://dx.doi.org/10.1016/j.iccl.2015.06.009
2211-7458/15/$ – see front matter © 2015 Elsevier Inc. All rights reserved.

(WSS).[2] Calculated as force per area (1 Pa = 1 N/m^2 = 10 dyne/cm^2), WSS is the parallel frictional force exerted on the arterial wall as blood flows past (Fig. 1). Blood flow and viscosity influence the WSS that is imparted onto the vessel surface and, as such, interplays between complex coronary geometry and dynamic blood flow produce variable hemodynamic WSS.[3]

The development of intravascular imaging has allowed for in vivo natural history investigations of the association between WSS and plaque development in patients with coronary artery disease. Computation of WSS in such patients (Fig. 2) begins during the cardiac catheterization procedure, in which patients ideally undergo coronary biplane angiography with intravascular imaging (either intravascular ultrasonography [IVUS] or optical coherence tomography) and Doppler flow velocity measurements. Meshed 3-dimensional geometries reconstructed from the fusion of intravascular imaging cross-sections and biplane angiographies are used in conjunction with patient-specific blood flow velocities to create computational fluid dynamic simulations and calculate WSS (Fig. 3). The accuracy of WSS computations depends on the level of detail that can be obtained regarding the patient's coronary anatomy and physiology.

Experimental studies and modeling paradigms have highlighted the importance of WSS magnitudes, particularly the impact of low WSS (<10 dyne/cm^2), on the development of endothelial dysfunction and atherosclerosis.

ROLE OF WALL SHEAR STRESS IN ENDOTHELIAL FUNCTION

Blood is transported to the myocardium through branching geometries of the coronary arterial system under pulsatile pressure. Coronary arterial flow is diastole dominant, dynamically complex, and spatiotemporally variable. The endothelium constitutes the critical contact surface between tissue and blood. Although physiologic variations of WSS influence endothelial-dependent acute changes of vascular tone and diameter, sustained abnormal WSS leads to the conversion of endothelial cells to a proatherogenic phenotype,[3,4] focal development of atherosclerosis, and adaptive vascular remodeling.[5,6] Endothelial function regulation by WSS can explain the focal propensity of atherosclerotic development in a milieu of systemic atherosclerosis risk factors.

MECHANOTRANSDUCTION OF WALL SHEAR STRESS IN ENDOTHELIAL CELLS

Endothelial cells sense WSS on their luminal side through primary cilia[7] and the glycocalyx, a highly charged glycoprotein-rich extension of the cell surface.[8] Subsequent intracellular transmission of hemodynamic shear stresses and resulting biochemical responses are depicted in Fig. 4 as the mechanotransduction of WSS.[3,9,10] The coupling of force to biochemical activity can occur simultaneously at multiple locations via the cytoskeleton, a central mediator in WSS signal crosstalk.[3] When exposed to oscillatory low WSS,

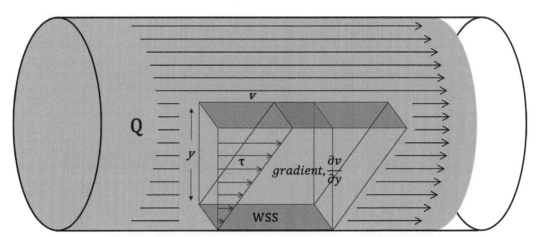

Fig. 1. Schematic of wall shear stress (WSS) in a coronary artery with blood flow. Blood flows through the vessel at a specific rate (Q). Expressed as force per unit area (eg, Pa), shear stress (τ) on the boundary surface (*gray parallelograms*) depends on the fluid velocity (v) at a specific distance from the boundary (y). WSS is τ along the vessel wall and is determined from both the gradient($\frac{\partial v}{\partial y}$) and blood viscosity.

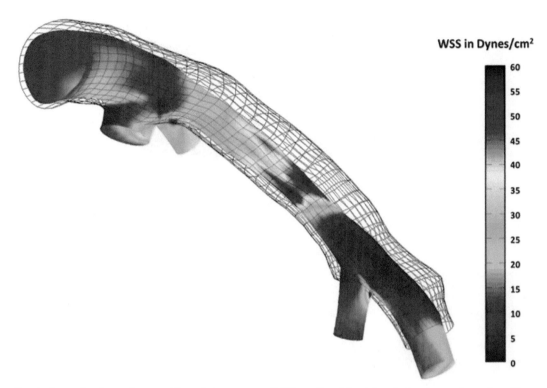

WSS in Dynes/cm²

Fig. 2. Example of a patient-specific wall shear stress (WSS) profile of the left anterior descending artery. Time-averaged WSS values (dynes/cm²) are circumferentially averaged for each intravascular ultrasound (IVUS) cross-section. The colors represent different WSS values as depicted in the scale. The outer mesh represents the external elastic membrane (EEM) and the area between the EEM and the lumen (*colored*) is considered to be plaque. Each cross-sectional line in the mesh represents 1 IVUS frame. (*From* Eshtehardi P, McDaniel MC, Suo J, et al. Association of coronary wall shear stress with atherosclerotic plaque burden, composition, and distribution in patients with coronary artery disease. J Am Heart Assoc 2012;1:e002543; with permission.)

both the mitogen-activated protein kinase and nuclear factor-κB signaling pathways become active and trigger phosphorylation cascades of signaling molecules and expression of procoagulant, proapoptotic, and proinflammatory genes that induce the atherosclerotic process.[11,12]

EFFECTS OF WALL SHEAR STRESS ON THE ENDOTHELIUM

Numerous in vitro and in vivo studies have shown that local WSS alterations can incite different endothelial cell morphologies and molecular responses in the initiation of atherosclerotic plaques (Table 1).

Endothelial Cell Phenotype

Physiologic WSS results in endothelial cell ellipsoidal morphology and alignment in the axial direction of blood flow; however, under low and oscillatory WSS, endothelial cells demonstrate an atherosusceptible phenotype with polygonal morphology and loss of alignment to blood flow.[13–15]

Low-density Lipoprotein Uptake

Low WSS increases the permeability of the endothelial cell surface to low-density lipoprotein cholesterol[16,17] and upregulates the expression of genes coding the low-density lipoprotein receptor, cholesterol synthase and fatty acid synthase.[18]

Nitric Oxide Production and Endothelial Nitric Oxide Synthase Expression

Nitric oxide is continuously synthesized from L-arginine in endothelial cells by the calcium-calmodulin–dependent enzyme endothelial nitric oxide synthase. Under physiologic condition, this enzyme plays a crucial role in maintaining normal endothelial function by modulating vasodilatory tone, regulating local cell growth, and protecting the vessel from injury.[19] Lower endothelial nitric oxide synthase expression has been observed in disturbed

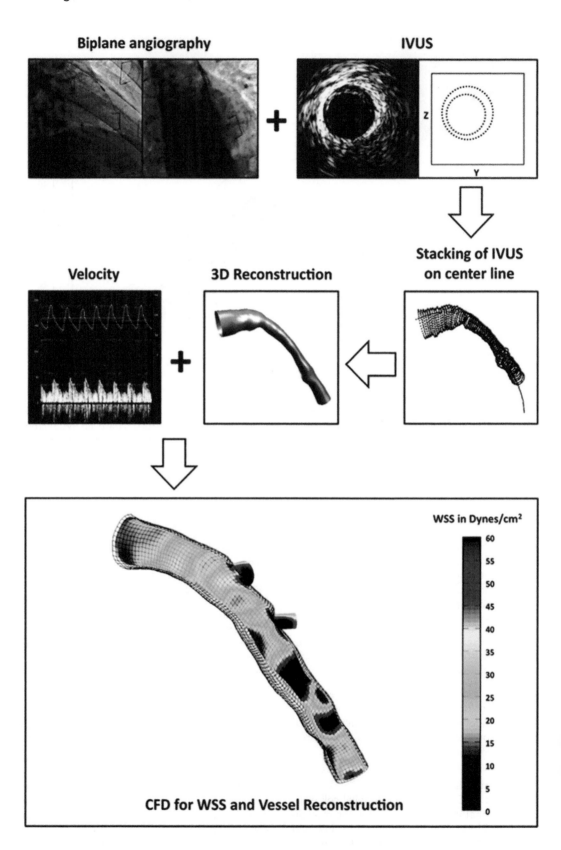

flow regions with low WSS compared with those with physiologic WSS.[5,20–22]

Oxidative Stress

Low WSS increases reactive oxygen species production via 3 mechanisms: (1) increased gene expression of major oxidative enzymes such as nicotinamide adenine dinucleotide phosphate and xanthine oxidases,[23–25] (2) endothelial nitric oxide synthase decoupling,[22,23] and (3) downregulation of intracellular ROS scavengers, such as manganese superoxide dismutase and glutathione.[11,26,27]

Proinflammatory Pathways

Regions of low WSS have high expressions of adhesion molecules, cytokines, chemoattractants and other inflammatory mediators[28–33] owing to enhanced proinflammatory gene expression through the mitogen-activated protein kinase and nuclear factor-κB pathways[34,35] and anti-inflammatory gene suppression from the Krüppel-like factor 2 and 4 (KLF-2/4) pathways.[36]

ROLE OF WALL SHEAR STRESS IN CORONARY PLAQUE PROGRESSION

Although atherosclerosis is a systemic chronic inflammatory disease, atherosclerotic plaques are not distributed uniformly throughout the vascular tree. Within coronary arteries, plaques are located frequently in areas of disturbed blood flow, such as arterial bifurcations and branch ostia (Fig. 5), where WSS is often determined to be low.[37,38] The temporal relationship between low WSS and plaque progression was first demonstrated in animal models, but studies have also shown this association to hold true in humans. Koskinas and colleagues[39] found that low WSS promoted plaque progression in a diabetic hyperlipidemic swine model of accelerated atherosclerosis. Excessive expansive remodeling, an exaggerated form of compensatory remodeling where both vessel and lumen dimensions increase, was observed in regions with marked plaque progression. This pattern of remodeling was found to reduce WSS, further driving plaque progression through continued lipid accumulation and inflammation. In a murine model, partial ligation of the carotid artery created patterns of low and oscillatory WSS, and these areas were associated with rapid atherosclerosis progression.[5] Interestingly, although low WSS is important in driving atherosclerosis, animal studies have shown that this mechanism seems to depend on cholesterol, with both atherogenic factors working synergistically to promote plaque growth (Fig. 6).[40]

Human studies confirm that low WSS is an essential factor in determining plaque progression. Stone and colleagues[41] demonstrated in 12 arteries that baseline low WSS regions were associated with plaque progression, as defined by an increase in IVUS plaque cross-sectional area. These results were confirmed by the same investigators in a larger patient cohort, with low WSS regions again exhibiting significant increases in plaque area and, in contrast to animal studies, constrictive remodeling.[6] Following this, Samady and colleagues[42] investigated the role of WSS in 20 patients undergoing virtual histology IVUS (VH-IVUS) at baseline and at 6 months of follow-up. Low baseline WSS regions developed increased plaque area at follow-up, along with an increase in VH-IVUS–defined necrotic core and fibrous tissue plaque components (Fig. 7). Consistent with previous longitudinal human studies, constrictive remodeling was observed more frequently in low WSS regions. Furthermore, WSS calculation, when compared with IVUS-based measures alone, provided incremental information for the prediction of plaque progression, including plaque burden.[43] Finally, in a serial IVUS study of 506 patients, Stone and colleagues[44] found that, compared with higher WSS areas, baseline low WSS regions were more likely to have increased plaque burden and constrictive remodeling at 6 to 10 months of follow-up.

Fig. 3. Schematic for the computation of patient-specific coronary arterial wall shear stress (WSS). Patients undergo cardiac catheterization with biplane angiography, intravascular ultrasound (IVUS) and Doppler flow velocity assessments. Reconstructed 3-dimensional vessel geometries are combined with patient-specific blood flow velocities to create computational fluid dynamic simulations and calculate WSS. The displayed results represent different WSS values (dynes/cm^2) as depicted on the scale. The outer mesh represents the external elastic membrane (EEM) and the area between the EEM and the lumen (*colored*) is considered to be plaque. Each cross-sectional line in the mesh represents 1 IVUS frame. (*From* Samady H, Eshtehardi P, McDaniel MC, et al. Coronary artery wall shear stress is associated with progression and transformation of atherosclerotic plaque and arterial remodeling in patients with coronary artery disease. Circulation 2011;124:781; with permission.)

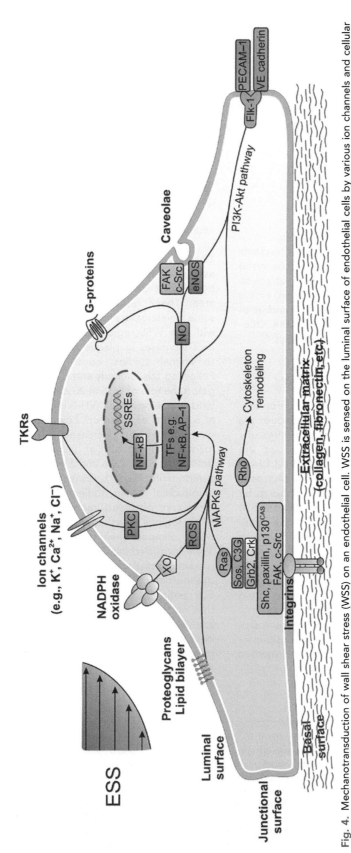

Fig. 4. Mechanotransduction of wall shear stress (WSS) on an endothelial cell. WSS is sensed on the luminal surface of endothelial cells by various ion channels and cellular receptors that activate integrins and adhesion molecules. This initiates several downstream signaling cascades that produce reactive oxygen species and activate mitogen-activated protein kinases (MAPKs) and other pathways, leading to cytoskeleton remodeling and phosphorylation of transcription factors such as nuclear factor (NF)-κB and Krüppel-like factor 2, which regulate expression of atherogenic or atheroprotective genes, respectively. AP-1, activator protein-1; eNOS, endothelial nitric oxide synthase; ESS, wall (endothelial) shear stress; FAK, focal adhesion kinase; NADPH, nicotinamide adenine dinucleotide phosphate; NO, nitric oxide; PECAM-1, platelet endothelial cell adhesion molecule-1; PI3K, phosphoinositide-3 kinase; PKC, protein kinase C; SSRE, shear stress responsive element; TF, transcription factor; TKR, tyrosine kinase receptor; VE, vascular endothelial; XO, xanthine oxidase. (From Chatzizisis YS, Coskun AU, Jonas M, et al. Role of endothelial shear stress in the natural history of coronary atherosclerosis and vascular behavior. J Am Coll Cardiol 2007;49:2385; with permission.)

Table 1	
Endothelial Response to Low WSS	
Feature	**Effects of Low WSS**
Endothelial cell morphology	Polygonal unaligned
Endothelial proliferation and apoptosis	Increased
Vasoactive agents	
Vasoconstrictors (ET-1/ECE, ACE)	Increased
Vasodilators (NO/eNOS, prostacyclin, CNP)	Decreased
Redox state	
Oxidative enzymes (NADPH oxidase, xanthine oxidase)	Increased
Antioxidant enzymes (Mn SOD, Cu/Zn SOD, glutathione)	Decreased
Growth regulators	
Growth promoters (PDGF-A, PDGF-B, ET-1, VEGF)	Increased
Growth inhibitors (NO/eNOS, TFG-β, PAI-1)	Decreased
Inflammation	
Chemoattractants (MCP-1)	Increased
Adhesion molecules (VCAM-1, ICAM-1, E-selectin)	Increased
Cytokines (TNF-α, IL-1, IFN-γ)	Increased
Thrombosis/fibrinolysis	
tPA	Decreased
NO/eNOS	Decreased
Endothelial LDL uptake, synthesis and permeability	Increased
Calcification (BMP-4)	Increased

Abbreviations: ACE, angiotensin-converting enzyme; BMP-4, bone morphogenic protein; CNP, C-type natriuretic peptide; Cu/Zn SOD, copper/zinc-containing superoxide dismutase; ECE, endothelin-converting enzyme; eNOS, endothelial nitric oxide synthase; ET-1, endothelin 1; ICAM-1, intracellular adhesion molecule-1; IFN-γ, interferon-γ; IL-1, interleukin-1; LDL, low-density lipoprotein cholesterol; MCP-1, monocyte chemotactic peptide 1; Mn SOD, manganese-containing superoxide dismutase; NADPH, nicotinamide adenine dinucleotide phosphate; NO, nitric oxide; PAI-1, plasminogen activator inhibitor-1; PDGF-A, B, platelet-derived growth factor A-chain, B-chain; TGF-β, transforming growth factor beta; TNF-α, tumor necrosis factor-α; tPA, tissue-type plasminogen activator; VCAM-1, vascular cell adhesion molecule 1; VEGF, vascular endothelial growth factor; WSS, wall shear stress.

Adapted from Malek AM, Alper SL, Izumo S. Hemodynamic shear stress and its role in atherosclerosis. JAMA 1999;282:2038, with permission; and Dhawan SS, Avati Nanjundappa RP, Branch JR, et al. Shear stress and plaque development. Expert Rev Cardiovasc Ther 2010;8:551, with permission.

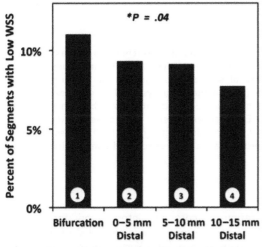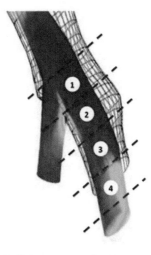

Fig. 5. Distribution of low wall shear stress (WSS) around bifurcations. (*Left*) Percentage of segments with low WSS within the bifurcations as well as at distances of 0 to 5 mm, 5 to 10, mm and 10 to 15 mm distal to bifurcations. (*Right*) On the WSS map, blue represents areas of low WSS. (*From* Eshtehardi P, McDaniel MC, Suo J, et al. Association of coronary wall shear stress with atherosclerotic plaque burden, composition, and distribution in patients with coronary artery disease. J Am Heart Assoc 2012;1:e002543; with permission.)

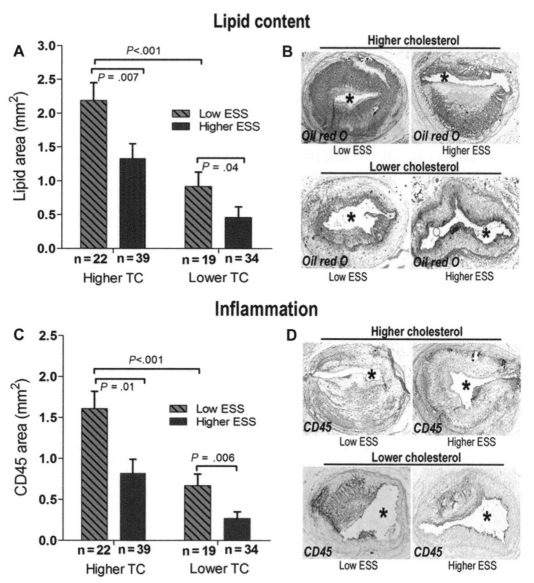

Fig. 6. Synergistic effect of wall shear stress (WSS) and systemic hypercholesterolemia on coronary atherosclerotic plaque progression and composition. (A) Quantitative analysis and (B) swine examples of oil-red-O staining demonstrating lipid accumulation in arterial segments categorized by higher versus lower systemic cholesterol levels and low versus greater WSS. (C) Quantitative analysis and (D) swine examples of CD45 immunostaining demonstrate leukocyte infiltration in arterial segments categorized by higher versus lower systemic cholesterol levels and low versus higher WSS. ESS, wall (endothelial) shear stress. * indicates the lumen. (*From* Koskinas KC, Chatzizisis YS, Papafaklis MI, et al. Synergistic effect of local endothelial shear stress and systemic hypercholesterolemia on coronary atherosclerotic plaque progression and composition in pigs. Int J Cardiol 2013;169:399; with permission.)

Decreased WSS was also found to be independently predictive of luminal obstruction at follow-up treated by percutaneous coronary intervention. This investigation is one of the few studies to associate WSS with clinical endpoints; however, the validity of percutaneous coronary intervention for worsening angiographic luminal obstruction remains controversial. Furthermore, combined WSS/IVUS assessment, with a positive predictive value of 41%, is currently not sufficiently robust for daily use in clinical practice.

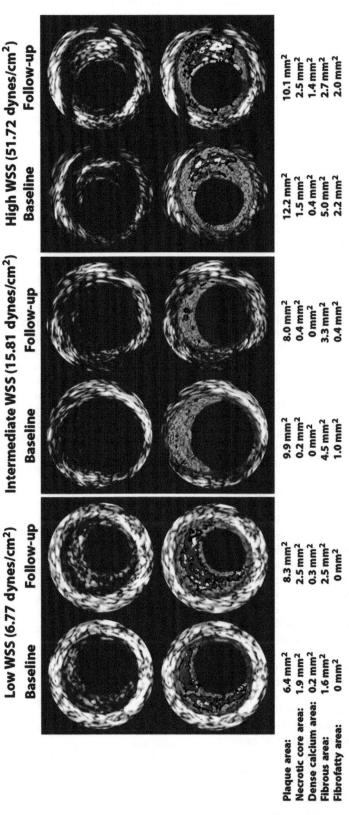

Fig. 7. Examples of intravascular ultrasound segments demonstrating plaque composition changes per baseline wall shear stress (WSS) categories. Plaque area and composition were assessed by virtual histology intravascular ultrasound and WSS was computed as described in Fig. 3. The low WSS segment demonstrates progression of plaque area, necrotic core area and fibrous area; the intermediate WSS segment demonstrates total plaque area regression; and the high WSS segment demonstrates total plaque area regression but progression of necrotic core and dense calcium areas. (*From* Samady H, Eshtehardi P, McDaniel MC, et al. Coronary artery wall shear stress is associated with progression and transformation of atherosclerotic plaque and arterial remodeling in patients with coronary artery disease. Circulation 2011;124:783; with permission.)

CORONARY PLAQUE TRANSFORMATION

Coronary plaques responsible for the majority of spontaneous thrombotic events exhibit large necrotic lipid cores, thin fibrous caps, presence of macrophages and evidence of intraplaque hemorrhage.[45] Although rupture is thought to occur when the structural stress within the plaque exceeds material strength,[46] alterations in WSS have been hypothesized as a potential mechanism that creates plaques vulnerable to failure.[47]

In animal studies, Cheng and colleagues[48] first observed that vascular regions with low WSS contained more lipid, less collagen and increased frequency of intraplaque hemorrhage. Their work was extended to the coronary tree by Chatzizisis and colleagues,[49] who conducted longitudinal swine studies and found that low WSS independently predicted the development of higher risk plaque phenotypes. These plaques displayed several features that create a rupture prone plaque substrate, including increased lipid accumulation, thinner fibrous caps, intense plaque inflammation and increased expression of matrix metalloproteinases, which act to reduce plaque strength through degradation of extracellular matrix proteins.[50] These adverse changes in plaque composition ultimately led to an increasing incidence of thin cap fibroatheromas in regions that were exposed to lower WSS.[51]

Assessing dynamic coronary plaque compositional changes in vivo has proven challenging because noninvasive imaging modalities fail to have sufficient resolution to reliably identify plaque components. However, several human studies have emerged that use intracoronary imaging to assess the effect of baseline WSS on temporal changes in plaque composition and classification. Using VH-IVUS, Wentzel and colleagues[52] found that necrotic core was located most frequently in low WSS regions during early atheroma formation and in high WSS regions in more advanced lesions. This bimodal association between WSS and necrotic core was also seen in 2 serial VH-IVUS studies, where increases in necrotic core area were observed both in low and high WSS regions, whereas calcification increased only in areas of high WSS.[42,43] Eshtehardi and colleagues[38] confirmed that, for every 10 dyne/cm^2 reduction in WSS, the percent necrotic core increased by approximately 17%, thus suggesting a connection between decreasing WSS and high-risk plaque transformation. Most recently, using optical coherence tomography, Vergallo and colleagues[53] found that low WSS regions had a higher prevalence of both lipid-rich plaques and optical coherence tomography-defined thin cap fibroatheromas. Additionally, fibrous cap thickness was reduced and macrophage density increased in low WSS regions, again implying a higher risk plaque phenotype. Finally, Gijsen and colleagues[54] found that high WSS regions colocalized with higher plaque structural strains, which may ultimately lead to plaque rupture.

SUMMARY

Coronary WSS computation has predominantly been used as a research tool; however, physicians have increasingly expressed interest in using WSS calculations in the clinical setting as image processing methods and computational power evolve. Low WSS offers incremental value in the prediction of atherosclerosis progression, especially in determining areas in the coronary vasculature that are more prone to develop vulnerable plaque morphologies. It may, therefore, be reasonable to consider low WSS regions in clinical decision making. Less well understood is the effect of high WSS on plaque development and transformation, specifically whether high WSS is a factor in excessive expansive remodeling and transformation to a higher risk plaque phenotype. Comprehensive prospective studies are needed to assess the utility of baseline WSS calculations on patient-specific outcomes, in the hope of identifying patients at the highest risk of clinical events.

REFERENCES

1. Krams R, Wentzel JJ, Oomen JA, et al. Evaluation of endothelial shear stress and 3D geometry as factors determining the development of atherosclerosis and remodeling in human coronary arteries in vivo. Combining 3D reconstruction from angiography and IVUS (ANGUS) with computational fluid dynamics. Arterioscler Thromb Vasc Biol 1997;17:2061–5.
2. Ku DN, Giddens DP, Zarins CK, et al. Pulsatile flow and atherosclerosis in the human carotid bifurcation. Positive correlation between plaque location and low oscillating shear stress. Arteriosclerosis 1985;5:293–302.
3. Davies PF. Hemodynamic shear stress and the endothelium in cardiovascular pathophysiology. Nat Clin Pract Cardiovasc Med 2009;6:16–26.
4. Davies PF, Civelek M, Fang Y, et al. The atherosusceptible endothelium: endothelial phenotypes in complex haemodynamic shear stress regions in vivo. Cardiovasc Res 2013;99:315–27.

5. Nam D, Ni CW, Rezvan A, et al. Partial carotid ligation is a model of acutely induced disturbed flow, leading to rapid endothelial dysfunction and atherosclerosis. Am J Physiol Heart Circ Physiol 2009;297:H1535–43.

6. Stone PH, Coskun AU, Kinlay S, et al. Regions of low endothelial shear stress are the sites where coronary plaque progresses and vascular remodelling occurs in humans: an in vivo serial study. Eur Heart J 2007;28:705–10.

7. Van der Heiden K, Hierck BP, Krams R, et al. Endothelial primary cilia in areas of disturbed flow are at the base of atherosclerosis. Atherosclerosis 2008; 196:542–50.

8. Weinbaum S, Tarbell JM, Damiano ER. The structure and function of the endothelial glycocalyx layer. Annu Rev Biomed Eng 2007;9:121–67.

9. Li YS, Haga JH, Chien S. Molecular basis of the effects of shear stress on vascular endothelial cells. J Biomech 2005;38:1949–71.

10. Chatzizisis YS, Coskun AU, Jonas M, et al. Role of endothelial shear stress in the natural history of coronary atherosclerosis and vascular remodeling: molecular, cellular, and vascular behavior. J Am Coll Cardiol 2007;49:2379–93.

11. Brooks AR, Lelkes PI, Rubanyi GM. Gene expression profiling of human aortic endothelial cells exposed to disturbed flow and steady laminar flow. Physiol Genomics 2002;9:27–41.

12. Dai G, Kaazempur-Mofrad MR, Natarajan S, et al. Distinct endothelial phenotypes evoked by arterial waveforms derived from atherosclerosis-susceptible and -resistant regions of human vasculature. Proc Natl Acad Sci U S A 2004;101:14871–6.

13. Levesque MJ, Nerem RM. The elongation and orientation of cultured endothelial cells in response to shear stress. J Biomech Eng 1985;107:341–7.

14. Levesque MJ, Liepsch D, Moravec S, et al. Correlation of endothelial cell shape and wall shear stress in a stenosed dog aorta. Arteriosclerosis 1986;6: 220–9.

15. Malek AM, Alper SL, Izumo S. Hemodynamic shear stress and its role in atherosclerosis. JAMA 1999; 282:2035–42.

16. Buchanan JR Jr, Kleinstreuer C, Truskey GA, et al. Relation between non-uniform hemodynamics and sites of altered permeability and lesion growth at the rabbit aorto-celiac junction. Atherosclerosis 1999;143:27–40.

17. Himburg HA, Grzybowski DM, Hazel AL, et al. Spatial comparison between wall shear stress measures and porcine arterial endothelial permeability. Am J Physiol Heart Circ Physiol 2004;286:H1916–22.

18. Goldstein JL, Kita T, Brown MS. Defective lipoprotein receptors and atherosclerosis. Lessons from an animal counterpart of familial hypercholesterolemia. N Engl J Med 1983;309:288–96.

19. Tousoulis D, Kampoli AM, Tentolouris C, et al. The role of nitric oxide on endothelial function. Curr Vasc Pharmacol 2012;10:4–18.

20. Ranjan V, Xiao Z, Diamond SL. Constitutive NOS expression in cultured endothelial cells is elevated by fluid shear stress. Am J Physiol 1995;269:H550–5.

21. Uematsu M, Ohara Y, Navas JP, et al. Regulation of endothelial cell nitric oxide synthase mRNA expression by shear stress. Am J Physiol 1995;269:C1371–8.

22. Won D, Zhu SN, Chen M, et al. Relative reduction of endothelial nitric-oxide synthase expression and transcription in atherosclerosis-prone regions of the mouse aorta and in an in vitro model of disturbed flow. Am J Pathol 2007;171:1691–704.

23. McNally JS, Davis ME, Giddens DP, et al. Role of xanthine oxidoreductase and NAD(P)H oxidase in endothelial superoxide production in response to oscillatory shear stress. Am J Physiol Heart Circ Physiol 2003;285:H2290–7.

24. Topper JN, Cai J, Falb D, et al. Identification of vascular endothelial genes differentially responsive to fluid mechanical stimuli: cyclooxygenase-2, manganese superoxide dismutase, and endothelial cell nitric oxide synthase are selectively up-regulated by steady laminar shear stress. Proc Natl Acad Sci U S A 1996;93:10417–22.

25. De Keulenaer GW, Chappell DC, Ishizaka N, et al. Oscillatory and steady laminar shear stress differentially affect human endothelial redox state: role of a superoxide-producing NADH oxidase. Circ Res 1998;82:1094–101.

26. Mueller CF, Widder JD, McNally JS, et al. The role of the multidrug resistance protein-1 in modulation of endothelial cell oxidative stress. Circ Res 2005; 97:637–44.

27. Inoue N, Ramasamy S, Fukai T, et al. Shear stress modulates expression of Cu/Zn superoxide dismutase in human aortic endothelial cells. Circ Res 1996; 79:32–7.

28. Shyy YJ, Hsieh HJ, Usami S, et al. Fluid shear stress induces a biphasic response of human monocyte chemotactic protein 1 gene expression in vascular endothelium. Proc Natl Acad Sci U S A 1994;91: 4678–82.

29. Suo J, Ferrara DE, Sorescu D, et al. Hemodynamic shear stresses in mouse aortas: implications for atherogenesis. Arterioscler Thromb Vasc Biol 2007;27:346–51.

30. Kawai Y, Matsumoto Y, Watanabe K, et al. Hemodynamic forces modulate the effects of cytokines on fibrinolytic activity of endothelial cells. Blood 1996;87:2314–21.

31. Sharefkin JB, Diamond SL, Eskin SG, et al. Fluid flow decreases preproendothelin mRNA levels and suppresses endothelin-1 peptide release in cultured human endothelial cells. J Vasc Surg 1991;14:1–9.

32. Masatsugu K, Itoh H, Chun TH, et al. Physiologic shear stress suppresses endothelin-converting enzyme-1 expression in vascular endothelial cells. J Cardiovasc Pharmacol 1998;31(Suppl 1):S42–5.

33. Ando J, Tsuboi H, Korenaga R, et al. Shear stress inhibits adhesion of cultured mouse endothelial cells to lymphocytes by downregulating VCAM-1 expression. Am J Physiol 1994;267:C679–87.

34. Hajra L, Evans AI, Chen M, et al. The NF-kappa B signal transduction pathway in aortic endothelial cells is primed for activation in regions predisposed to atherosclerotic lesion formation. Proc Natl Acad Sci U S A 2000;97:9052–7.

35. Passerini AG, Polacek DC, Shi C, et al. Coexisting proinflammatory and antioxidative endothelial transcription profiles in a disturbed flow region of the adult porcine aorta. Proc Natl Acad Sci U S A 2004;101:2482–7.

36. Dekker RJ, van Soest S, Fontijn RD, et al. Prolonged fluid shear stress induces a distinct set of endothelial cell genes, most specifically lung Kruppel-like factor (KLF2). Blood 2002;100:1689–98.

37. Dhawan SS, Avati Nanjundappa RP, Branch JR, et al. Shear stress and plaque development. Expert Rev Cardiovasc Ther 2010;8:545–56.

38. Eshtehardi P, McDaniel MC, Suo J, et al. Association of coronary wall shear stress with atherosclerotic plaque burden, composition, and distribution in patients with coronary artery disease. J Am Heart Assoc 2012;1:e002543.

39. Koskinas KC, Feldman CL, Chatzizisis YS, et al. Natural history of experimental coronary atherosclerosis and vascular remodeling in relation to endothelial shear stress: a serial, in vivo intravascular ultrasound study. Circulation 2010;121:2092–101.

40. Koskinas KC, Chatzizisis YS, Papafaklis MI, et al. Synergistic effect of local endothelial shear stress and systemic hypercholesterolemia on coronary atherosclerotic plaque progression and composition in pigs. Int J Cardiol 2013;169:394–401.

41. Stone PH, Coskun AU, Kinlay S, et al. Effect of endothelial shear stress on the progression of coronary artery disease, vascular remodeling, and in-stent restenosis in humans: in vivo 6-month follow-up study. Circulation 2003;108:438–44.

42. Samady H, Eshtehardi P, McDaniel MC, et al. Coronary artery wall shear stress is associated with progression and transformation of atherosclerotic plaque and arterial remodeling in patients with coronary artery disease. Circulation 2011;124:779–88.

43. Corban MT, Eshtehardi P, Suo J, et al. Combination of plaque burden, wall shear stress, and plaque phenotype has incremental value for prediction of coronary atherosclerotic plaque progression and vulnerability. Atherosclerosis 2014;232:271–6.

44. Stone PH, Saito S, Takahashi S, et al. Prediction of progression of coronary artery disease and clinical outcomes using vascular profiling of endothelial shear stress and arterial plaque characteristics: the PREDICTION Study. Circulation 2012;126:172–81.

45. Virmani R, Kolodgie FD, Burke AP, et al. Lessons from sudden coronary death: a comprehensive morphological classification scheme for atherosclerotic lesions. Arterioscler Thromb Vasc Biol 2000;20:1262–75.

46. Teng Z, Brown AJ, Calvert PA, et al. Coronary plaque structural stress is associated with plaque composition and subtype and higher in acute coronary syndrome: the BEACON I (Biomechanical Evaluation of Atheromatous Coronary Arteries) study. Circ Cardiovasc Imaging 2014;7:461–70.

47. Pedrigi RM, de Silva R, Bovens SM, et al. Thin-cap fibroatheroma rupture is associated with a fine interplay of shear and wall stress. Arterioscler Thromb Vasc Biol 2014;34:2224–31.

48. Cheng C, Tempel D, van Haperen R, et al. Atherosclerotic lesion size and vulnerability are determined by patterns of fluid shear stress. Circulation 2006;113:2744–53.

49. Chatzizisis YS, Jonas M, Coskun AU, et al. Prediction of the localization of high-risk coronary atherosclerotic plaques on the basis of low endothelial shear stress: an intravascular ultrasound and histopathology natural history study. Circulation 2008;117:993–1002.

50. Chatzizisis YS, Baker AB, Sukhova GK, et al. Augmented expression and activity of extracellular matrix-degrading enzymes in regions of low endothelial shear stress colocalize with coronary atheromata with thin fibrous caps in pigs. Circulation 2011;123:621–30.

51. Koskinas KC, Sukhova GK, Baker AB, et al. Thin-capped atheromata with reduced collagen content in pigs develop in coronary arterial regions exposed to persistently low endothelial shear stress. Arterioscler Thromb Vasc Biol 2013;33:1494–504.

52. Wentzel JJ, Schuurbiers JC, Gonzalo Lopez N, et al. In vivo assessment of the relationship between shear stress and necrotic core in early and advanced coronary artery disease. EuroIntervention 2013;9:989–95 [discussion: 995].

53. Vergallo R, Papafaklis MI, Yonetsu T, et al. Endothelial shear stress and coronary plaque characteristics in humans: a combined frequency-domain optical coherence tomography and computational fluid dynamics study. Circ Cardiovasc Imaging 2014;7:905–11.

54. Gijsen FJ, Wentzel JJ, Thury A, et al. Strain distribution over plaques in human coronary arteries relates to shear stress. Am J Physiol Heart Circ Physiol 2008;295:H1608–14.

Moving?

Make sure your subscription moves with you!

To notify us of your new address, find your **Clinics Account Number** (located on your mailing label above your name), and contact customer service at:

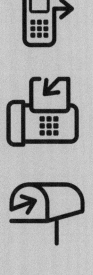

Email: journalscustomerservice-usa@elsevier.com

800-654-2452 (subscribers in the U.S. & Canada)
314-447-8871 (subscribers outside of the U.S. & Canada)

Fax number: 314-447-8029

Elsevier Health Sciences Division
Subscription Customer Service
3251 Riverport Lane
Maryland Heights, MO 63043

ELSEVIER

Printed and bound by CPI Group (UK) Ltd, Croydon, CR0 4YY

03/10/2024

01040377-0005